Handbook for Synthesizing
Qualitative Research

About the Authors

MARGARETE SANDELOWSKI, PhD, RN, FAAN, is Cary C. Boshamer Distinguished Professor at the University of North Carolina at Chapel Hill (UNC-CH) School of Nursing and principal investigator of the Qualitative Metasynthesis Project on which this book is based. She is also director of the Annual Summer Institute in Qualitative Research held at UNC-CH School of Nursing. Dr. Sandelowski is one of three associate editors of *Research in Nursing & Health,* and a member of the editorial boards of *Advances in Nursing Science, Field Methods, Journal of Mixed Methods Research, Nursing Inquiry,* and *Qualitative Health Research.* She is internationally recognized for her expertise in qualitative methods. She has more than 120 publications in both nursing and social science journals and books, with over 35 refereed papers on qualitative methods alone. The ethnographic work, *With Child in Mind: Studies of the Personal Encounter With Infertility* (1993), was awarded a national book prize from the American Anthropological Association. *Devices and Desires: Gender, Technology, and American Nursing* (2000), a social history of technology in nursing, has been favorably reviewed in both nursing and medical history journals.

JULIE BARROSO, PhD, ANP, APRN, BC, is associate professor and director of the Adult Nurse Practitioner Program at Duke University School of Nursing, and co-principal investigator of the Qualitative Metasynthesis Project. She is also a senior research fellow with the Health Inequalities Program (part of the Terry Sanford Institute of Public Policy at Duke University) and served as chair of the Research Committee, part of the National Leadership Council for the Association of Nurses in AIDS Care. Her practice, research, and teaching have focused on people with HIV infection. Dr. Barroso has conducted both qualitative and quantitative research in this area, including a metasynthesis of studies with HIV-positive men, study of physiological and psychological correlates of fatigue, a psychometric study of the HIV-Related Fatigue Scale, and a secondary analysis of a 12-year longitudinal data set to examine the relationship between fatigue and depression in HIV-positive gay men. She is currently principal investigator of a National Institute of Nursing Research longitudinal study of physiological, psychosocial, and personal factors in the development of HIV-related fatigue. Dr. Barroso maintains a practice at the Duke University AIDS Research and Treatment Center.

Handbook for Synthesizing Qualitative Research

MARGARETE SANDELOWSKI, PhD, RN, FAAN
JULIE BARROSO, PhD, ANP, APRN, BC

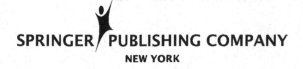

SPRINGER PUBLISHING COMPANY
NEW YORK

Springer Publishing Company, Inc.
11 West 42nd Street
New York, NY 10036

Acquisitions Editor: Sally J. Barhydt
Production Editor: Sara Yoo
Cover design by Joanne E. Honigman
Typeset by Daily Information Processing, Churchville, PA

06 07 08 09 10 / 5 4 3 2 1

Library of Congress Cataloging-in-Publication Data

Sandelowski, Margarete.
    Handbook for synthesizing qualitative research / by Margarete Sandelowski and Julie Barroso.
        p. ; cm.
    Includes bibliographical references and index.
    ISBN 0-8261-5694-0
    1. Qualitative research. 2. Medicine—Research—Methodology.
I. Barroso, Julie. II. Title.
    [DNLM: 1. Qualitative Research. 2. Biomedical Research.
W 20.5 S214h 2006]

R853.Q34S26   2006
610.72—dc22
                                                          2006009077

Printed in the United States of America by Bang Printing.

Contents

Preface

Welcome to the *Handbook for Synthesizing Qualitative Research*, a guide for integrating the findings in reports of primary qualitative studies. Qualitative research synthesis is scientific inquiry aimed at systematically reviewing and formally integrating the findings in reports of completed qualitative studies. The phrase *qualitative research synthesis* refers both to an interpretive product (i.e., the synthesis itself, or integration of a set of findings) and to the methods and techniques used to create that product (i.e., the processes involved in producing a synthesis). Written for graduate nursing students and faculty, as well as students and faculty in other healthcare and practice disciplines, this handbook will help you:

1. Locate qualitative research synthesis in the contemporary landscape of qualitative research, research synthesis, research utilization, and evidence-based practice;
2. Locate the qualitative research synthesis enterprise in reading and writing practices;
3. Differentiate qualitative research synthesis from other forms of inquiry;
4. Formulate significant research problems and purposes for a qualitative research synthesis study;
5. Design credible qualitative research synthesis studies that fit available resources;
6. Conduct comprehensive searches for primary qualitative research reports in a target domain of inquiry;
7. Conduct judicious appraisals of these qualitative research reports;
8. Compare and classify the findings across these qualitative research reports;
9. Select methodological approaches appropriate to the content and form of the qualitative research findings in these reports;

10. Use qualitative metasummary and metasynthesis techniques to integrate qualitative research findings;
11. Optimize the validity of qualitative research synthesis studies; and
12. Present the results of qualitative research synthesis studies in effective, audience-appropriate ways.

In this *Handbook,* we illustrate procedures for conducting qualitative research synthesis projects with reports of studies in two domains of research: qualitative studies conducted with HIV-positive women and with women and couples who received positive prenatal diagnoses. These reports represent research across the behavioral and social science and practice disciplines, including anthropology, psychology, sociology, nursing, and public health. They also represent our respective areas of expertise. Reviewers generally choose topics for research synthesis in areas in which they have expertise and to which they have strong commitments. We use these reports to describe methods that were clarified, refined, or newly developed in the course of the National Institutes of Health, National Institute of Nursing Research study we conducted, entitled *Analytic Techniques for Qualitative Metasynthesis* (R01NR04907 & R01NR04907S, 06/01/2000–06/02/2005). You can read an annotated version of the proposal for this study in Sandelowski & Barroso (2003). The Web site for this Project is available at http://www.unc.edu/~msandelo/qmp/. We refer to this study throughout this book as the Metasynthesis Project.

The sample of HIV studies we draw from here consists of 114 reports appearing between 1991 (the year of the first study known to us to meet our inclusion criteria) and 2002, including 79 published reports (75 journal articles, 2 books, 1 book chapter, and 1 technical report) and 35 unpublished reports (31 doctoral dissertations and 4 master's theses). These works were retrieved between June 1, 2000, and December 31, 2002. The sample of positive prenatal diagnosis studies consists of 17 reports appearing between 1984 (the year of the first study known to us to meet our inclusion criteria) and 2002, including 13 published reports (10 journal articles, 2 books, and 1 book chapter) and 4 unpublished reports (3 doctoral dissertations and 1 master's thesis). These reports were retrieved between December 1, 2002, and March 31, 2003. All of these reports are listed in the Appendix.

To facilitate your understanding of several of the processes involved in transforming research findings into research syntheses, we created a web site to illustrate them in a more dynamic visual form. At this site, you will find materials to supplement Chapters 3, 4, and 6. Please visit http://www.unc.edu/~msandelo/handbook whenever we refer you to it in the book.

We are pleased that you are considering this *Handbook* for your work. We hope that you will find in it the assistance you need to conduct your qualitative research synthesis project.

MARGARETE SANDELOWSKI
JULIE BARROSO

REFERENCE

Sandelowski, M., & Barroso, J. (2003). Writing the proposal for a qualitative research methodology project. *Qualitative Health Research, 13,* 781–820.

Acknowledgments

This book and the research on which it is based were made possible by two grants from the National Institute of Nursing Research/National Institutes of Health (R01NR04907 & R01NR04907S) for the study *Analytic Techniques for Qualitative Metasynthesis.* We thank the following: Sandy Funk, associate dean for research and director of the Research Support Center at the University of North Carolina at Chapel Hill School of Nursing, whose incisive critique, tireless efforts, and generous spirit contributed to the success of the proposal for this project; the anonymous grant reviewers who were willing to make the leap of faith that made this project possible and whose critiques helped us improve its value as scholarship; and Martha Hare, of the National Institute of Nursing Research, for her unfailing support.

We also gratefully acknowledge the scholars who served as members of the expert panel for this project: Cheryl T. Beck of the University of Connecticut; Louise Jensen of the University of Alberta; Margaret Kearney of the University of Rochester; George Noblit of the University of North Carolina at Chapel Hill School of Education; Gail Powell-Cope of the University of South Florida and James A. Haley Veterans Affairs Medical Center in Tampa, Florida; and Sally Thorne of the University of British Columbia. Their diligence, generosity, and humor in doing their "homework" for the project and participating in our lively panel meetings helped us keep our eyes on the prize.

We are also most grateful to Jennifer D'Auria and Miriam Jicha at the University of North Carolina at Chapel Hill School of Nursing, and Mark Koyanagi (formerly of that institution), for their artistry and expertise in instructional technology and web and information design. Jennifer and Mark designed and executed the innovative online supplement to this book, referred to in the preface, and Miriam designed the illustrations in this book.

We thank Claudia Gollop of the University of North Carolina at Chapel Hill School of Information and Library Science; Linda Collins, Lynne Morris, Julia Shaw-Kokot, and K. T. L. Vaughan of the User Services Department at the University of North Carolina at Chapel Hill Health Sciences Library; and Anne D. Powers of the Duke University Medical Center Library for their expertise in information science and technology. And, we salute the graduate students—including April Edlin, Camille Lambe, Janet Meynell, Oknam Park, and Patricia Pearce—who have served this project so well as research assistants.

Last, but never least, we offer a most appreciative nod to the University of North Carolina at Chapel Hill itself for providing such a vibrant and hospitable professional home for our work.

Permissions to Publish

This book contains material in a revised form previously published, by permission of:

ASSOCIATION OF WOMEN'S HEALTH, OBSTETRIC AND NEONATAL NURSES

Sandelowski, M., & Barroso, J. (2005). The travesty of choosing after positive prenatal diagnosis. *JOGNN: Journal of Obstetric, Gynecologic, and Neonatal Nursing, 34* 307–318.

AUTHOR

Sandelowski, M. (2006). "Meta-jeopardy": The crisis of representation in qualitative metasynthesis. *Nursing Outlook, 54,* 10–16.
Sandelowski, M., & Barroso, J. (2002). Reading qualitative studies. *International Journal of Qualitative Methods, 1*(1), Article 5. On line journal available at http://www.ualberta.ca/~ijqm/english/engframeset.html

BLACKWELL

Sandelowski, M., Lambe, C., & Barroso, J. (2004). Stigma in HIV-positive women. *Journal of Nursing Scholarship, 36,* 122–128.
Siegel K., & Schrimshaw, E. W. (2001). Reasons and justifications for considering pregnancy among women living with HIV/AIDS. *Psychology of Women Quarterly, 25,* 112–123.

LIPPINCOTT WILLIAMS & WILKINS

Sandelowski, M., & Barroso, J. (2003). Creating metasummaries of qualitative findings. *Nursing Research, 52,* 226–233.

SAGE

Barroso, J., Gollop, C. J., Sandelowski, M., Meynell, J., Pearce, P. F., & Collins, L. J. (2003). The challenges of searching for and retrieving qualitative studies. *Western Journal of Nursing Research, 25,* 153–178.

Sandelowski, M. (2003). Tables or tableaux? Writing and reading mixed methods studies. In A. Tashakkori & C. Teddlie (Eds.), *Handbook of mixed methods in social and behavioral research* (pp. 321–350). Thousand Oaks, CA: Sage.

Sandelowski, M., & Barroso, J. (2003). Classifying the findings in qualitative studies. *Qualitative Health Research, 13,* 905–923.

WILEY

Sandelowski, M., & Barroso, J. (2003). Motherhood in the context of maternal HIV infection. *Research in Nursing & Health, 26,* 470–482.

Sandelowski, M., & Barroso, J. (2003). Toward a metasynthesis of qualitative findings on motherhood in HIV-positive women. *Research in Nursing & Health, 26,* 153–170.

Introduction:
Attitudes, Assumptions, and Caveats

We intend for you to use this *Handbook* as a methodological toolbox and as a stimulus to thinking and creativity, not as a prescriptive set of rules and procedures to be rigidly followed. Methodological prescriptions impede the methodological innovation, imaginative analysis, and interpretation required to conduct qualitative research synthesis studies. Without violating method assumptions or imperatives, you should accommodate methods to your study, not your study to methods. Qualitative research synthesis projects require methodological craftsmanship, not "methodolatry" or methodological "purity." These projects also demand that reviewers address persistent challenges and controversies in conducting research synthesis studies in general, and in qualitative research in particular, and, therefore, a broad understanding of both qualitative research and research synthesis is required.

Synthesizing qualitative research is an inescapably iterative and dynamic process, as the outcomes of work in each phase of study will compel you to rethink the work completed in previous phases. Indeed, you will find yourself resetting study boundaries, redefining key terms, revising procedures, and generally remaking decisions throughout the life of your project. Accordingly, if there are any methodological "rules" to be adhered to, they are:

1. Accommodate methods to your study in ways that violate neither their philosophical foundations nor the integrity of the reports in your study;
2. Be flexible yet systematic; and
3. Account for and clarify all the judgments you make.

By following these rules, you will be in a position to preserve the qualitative research attitude of reflexivity and critique and the emergent nature of qualitative research design and to avoid misrepresenting researchers' findings and the research participants' experiences from which these findings derive.

Findings Thrice Removed

An important caveat to the qualitative research synthesis enterprise described in this *Handbook* is that it inescapably consists of reviewers' constructions of researchers' constructions of the data they obtained from research participants, which are themselves constructed within the research encounter. (To avoid confusion, we use the term *researchers* in this book to refer to the scholars who conducted the primary studies and who authored the reports of those studies included in qualitative research synthesis projects. We use the term *reviewers* to refer to the scholars conducting qualitative research synthesis studies.) From the vantage point of the reviewer (i.e., you), the actors whose points of view are the targets of qualitative research synthesis studies are the researchers/authors who created/reported the findings. The research findings from primary qualitative studies—the primary data in qualitative research synthesis studies—are researchers' representations of the experiences told to them by research participants; they are, thus, told experiences retold.

Qualitative research syntheses are, therefore, at the very least, three times removed from the lived experiences of the research participants they are meant to represent. Qualitative research synthesis is inescapably an act of re-presenting representations. Indeed, the qualitative research synthesis enterprise troubles the line between reality and representation as reviewers' only access to the experiences of research participants is through the representations of researchers in their reports. The qualitative research synthesis enterprise thereby holds the potential to intensify the "crisis of representation" (Smith, 2004) that continues to be a central concern in the qualitative research community. Central to this crisis is the challenge to the assumption that any human-subjects inquiry can ever faithfully and fairly represent the lives of those subjects. When the research purpose is to synthesize research findings, the problem of representation is potentially increased exponentially (Sandelowski, 2006). Reviewers conducting qualitative research synthesis projects must, therefore, assume a methodologically self-conscious stance whereby they show their awareness of the wide gap that may exist between the lived experiences depicted in research reports and their own interpretive integrations of them. We further consider issues relating to representation in qualitative research synthesis throughout this book, but especially in chapter 9.

Continuing our thematic emphasis on the blurred line between representation and reality in qualitative research synthesis is our focus on reports, as opposed to studies. In research synthesis projects, you are not reviewing studies per se, but rather the reports of those studies. Research reports are after-the-fact reconstructions of studies, not the studies themselves; they are accounts of studies, not mirror reflections of them. Reports are intended to make readers "virtual . . . (yet) trusting witnesses" to studies, the conduct of which they cannot actually observe in the flesh (Shapin, 1984, pp. 490–491). Research reports are dynamic vehicles that mediate between the researchers who wrote them and the reviewers who read them. That makes research synthesis studies not only a scientific, but also a literary enterprise demanding a wide-ranging knowledge of scientific and ethnographic rhetoric and representation. Our focus in this book on reporting style and form is meant to emphasize the inseparability of form from content and the unavoidable fact that all texts—including scientific ones—are clothed in literary garments (Ayres & Poirier, 1996). Researchers write their reports to conform to stylistic conventions for writing up scientific reports. Style is, therefore, not a frill, but rather an embodiment of content. How researchers/authors are expected to write affects and even constrains what they write and, therefore, shapes what is taken to be knowledge (Richardson, 2000).

Reviewers/readers of research reports bring to these texts a dynamic and unique configuration of experiences, knowledge, personality traits, and sociocultural orientations. Fish (1980) proposed that readers belong to one or more "interpretive communities" (e.g., qualitative researchers, academic nurses, social constructionists) that strongly influence how they read, why they read, and what they read into any one text. The members of these communities differ in their access and attunement to, knowledge and acceptance of, and participation with, for example, references and allusions in a text, the varied uses of words and numbers, and various genres or conventions of writing. Because of their varying reading backgrounds, experiences, and expectations, readers will vary in their interaction with texts (Beach, 1993; Lye, 1996a, b). Even when one reader is engaged with the same text, interactions will vary, as such factors as the passage of time and different reasons for reading that text will alter the reading. Moreover, reading is cumulative as each new reading builds upon preceding readings of this and other texts (Manguel, 1996).

Researchers/writers, in turn, employ various writing conventions and literary devices in order to appeal to readers, and to shape and control their readings. Shape is a property of information that includes, not just the informational content per se, but also the very physical form in which it appears (Dillon & Vaughan, 1997). Indeed, the research report is itself better viewed, not as an end-stage write-up, but rather as a dynamic—"literary technology"—(Shapin, 1984) whereby writers use literary devices—such as correlation coefficients and p values in reports of quantitative research, and quotations, metaphors, and coding schemas in reports of qualitative research—to engage readers rhetorically to accept their study procedures and findings as valid. Researchers/writers "deploy . . . (these) linguistic resources" (Shapin, 1984, p. 491) to appeal to different communities of scholars. In the case of the correlation coefficient, the appeal is to stability and consensus; in the case of the quotation, the appeal is to "giving voice." These devices contribute to the illusion that write-ups of research are reflections of reality and that readers are actually witnessing the study reported there.

Statistics are not merely numeric transformations of data, but also "literary . . . displays treated as dramatic presentations to a scientific community" (Gephart, 1988, p. 47). In quantitative research, the appeal to numbers gives studies their rhetorical power. Statistics are a naturalized and rule-governed means of producing what is perceived to be the most conclusive knowledge about a target phenomenon (John, 1992). John (1992, p. 146) proposed that statistics confer the "epistemic authority" of science. The power of statistics lies as much in their ability to engender a "sense of conviction" (John, 1992, p. 147) in their "evidentiary value" (p. 144) as to provide actual evidence about a target phenomenon. Statistics play a dramatic role authorizing the science in the "artful literary display" (Gephart, 1988, p. 63) known as the scientific report, and they are a means to create meaning. Writers do not find, so much as they participate with willing readers to create, quantitative significance (Gephart, 1986). Communities of scholars are created and sustained by virtue of this participation (Clark, 1990).

Whereas tables and figures provide much of the appeal in quantitative research, tableaux of experience and figures of speech provide much of the appeal in qualitative research. Writers wanting to write appealing qualitative research reports tend to use devices, such as expressive language, quotations, and case descriptions, in order to communicate that they have recognized and managed well the tensions, paradoxes, and contradictions of qualitative inquiry. Qualitative writers desire to tell "tales of the field" (Van Maanen, 1988) that convey methodological rigor, but also methodological flexibility; their ability to achieve intimacy with, but also to maintain their distance from, their subjects and data; and, their fidelity to the tenets of objective inquiry, but also their feeling for the persons and events they observed. They want their reports to be as true as science is commonly held to be, and yet as evocative as art is supposed to be.

In summary, the only site for evaluating research studies—whether they are qualitative or quantitative—is the report itself. The "production of knowledge" cannot be separated from the "communication of knowledge" by which "communities" of responsive readers are created and then come to accept a study as valid (Shapin, 1984, p. 481). Debates about validity are, therefore, as much about rhetoric and representation as they are about "truth." The production of convincing findings lies at least as much (if not more) in how well they meet the expectations of readers representing a variety of interpretive communities as it does in the correspondence of these findings to actual events or "reality." Indeed, although a line is typically drawn between epistemic and aesthetic criteria, they are in practice components of each other. The sense of rightness and feeling of comfort readers experience reading the report of a study constitute the very judgments they make about the validity or trustworthiness of the study itself. All forms"whether novel, pottery, or scientific report"are evaluated by the same aesthetic criteria, including coherence, attractiveness, and economy (Eisner, 1985). Quantification and graphical displays are common ways to achieve these goals in quantitative research reports (Law & Whittaker, 1988), while conceptual renderings, quotations, and narratives are common ways to achieve these goals in qualitative research reports. The aesthetic is itself a "mode of knowing" (Eisner, 1985), whereby both scientific and artistic forms are judged by how well they confer order and stimulate the senses.

Accordingly, whether you—as a reviewer—judge a set of research findings as vivid or lifeless, coherent or confusing, novel or pedestrian, or as ringing true or false, you are ultimately making, not just a communal judgment, but also a uniquely personal and aesthetic one (Bochner, 2000; Lynch & Edgerton, 1988; Richardson, 2000). Although reviewers of scientific reports typically hold the search for truth as a "regulative ideal" (Murphy & Dingwall, 2001, p. 346), their "readings" of studies are key shapers of the truths/syntheses they produce.

REFERENCES

Ayres, L., & Poirier, S. (1996). Virtual text and the growth of meaning in qualitative analysis. *Research in Nursing & Health, 19,* 163–169.

Beach, R. (1993). *A teacher's introduction to reader-response theories.* Urbana, IL: National Council of Teachers of English.

Bochner, A. P. (2000). Criteria against ourselves. *Qualitative Inquiry, 6,* 266–272.

Clark, G. (1990). *Dialogue, dialectic, and conversation: A social perspective on the function of writing.* Carbondale: Southern Illinois University Press.

Dillon, A., & Vaughan, M. (1997). "It's the journey and the destination":

Shape and the emergent property of genre in evaluating digital documents. *New Review of Multimedia and Hypermedia, 3,* 91–106.

Eisner, E. (1985). Aesthetic modes of knowing. In E. Eisner (Ed.), *Learning and teaching the ways of knowing: Eighty-fourth yearbook of the National Society for the study of education, Part II* (pp. 23–36). Chicago: National Society of the Study of Education.

Fish, S. (1980). *Is there a text in this class? The authority of interpretive communities.* Cambridge, MA: Harvard University Press.

Gephart, R. P. (1986). Deconstructing the defense for quantification in social science: A content analysis of journal articles on the parametric strategy. *Qualitative Sociology, 9,* 126–144.

Gephart, R. P. (1988). *Ethnostatistics: Qualitative foundations for quantitative research.* Beverly Hills, CA: Sage.

John, I. D. (1992). Statistics as rhetoric in psychology. *Australian Psychologist, 27,* 144–149.

Law, J., & Whittaker, J. (1988). On the art of representation: Notes on the politics of visualization. In G. Fyfe & J. Law (Eds.), *Picturing power: Visual depiction and social relations* (pp. 160–183). London: Routledge.

Lye, J. (1996a). *Reader-response: Various positions.* Retrieved July 5, 2004, from www.brocku.ca/english/courses/4F70/rr.html

Lye, J. (1996b). *Some factors affecting/effecting the reading of texts.* Retrieved July 5, 2004, from http://www.brocku.ca/english/courses/4F70/factors.html

Lynch, M., & Edgerton, S. Y. (1988). Aesthetics and digital image processing: Representational craft in contemporary astronomy. In G. Fyfe & J. Law (Eds.), *Picturing power: Visual depiction and social relations* (pp. 184–220). London: Routledge.

Manguel, A. (1996). *A history of reading.* Toronto: Alfred A. Knopf.

Murphy, E. & Dingwall, R. (2001). The ethics of ethnography. In P. Atkinson, A. Coffey, S. Delamont, J. Lofland, & L. Lofland (Eds.), *Handbook of ethnography* (pp. 339–351). London: Sage.

Richardson, L. (2000). Writing: A method of inquiry. In N. K. Denzin & Y. S. Lincoln (Eds.), *Handbook of qualitative research* (2nd ed; pp. 923–948). Thousand Oaks, CA: Sage.

Sandelowski, M. (2006). "Meta-Jeopardy": The crisis of representation in qualitative metasynthesis. *Nursing Outlook, 54,* 10–16.

Shapin, S. (1984). Pump and circumstance: Robert Boyle's literary technology. *Social Studies of Science, 14,* 481–520.

Smith, J. K. (2004). Representation, crisis of. In M. S. Lewis-Beck, A. Bryman, & T. F. Liao (Eds.), *The Sage encyclopedia of social science research methods* (Vol. 3, pp. 962–963). Thousand Oaks, CA: Sage.

Van Maanen, J. (1988). *Tales of the field: On writing ethnography.* Chicago: University of Chicago Press.

List of Tables, Figures, and Boxes

TABLES

Chapter 6

Chapter 7

Chapter 8

Chapter 9

FIGURES

Chapter 1

BOXES

Quotations

Methods are tools for the production of knowledge (A. E. Clarke, *Situational analysis: Grounded theory after the postmodern turn.* Thousand Oaks, CA: Sage, 2005, p. 304).

Methods are not a way of opening a window on the world, but a way of interfering with it (A. Mol, *The body multiple: Ontology in medical practice.* Durham, NC: Duke University Press, 2002, p. 155).

Truth can be a synthesis, or an impression (S. Hazzard, *The great fire.* New York: Picador, 2003, p. 46).

The only thing that links them together is you. You are their thread (J. Carroll, *The marriage of sticks.* New York: Tor, 1999, p. 215).

She taught me not how to reassemble, but how to rearrange (T. Greenwood, *Undressing the moon.* New York: St. Martin's Press, 2002, p. 241).

CHAPTER ONE

The Urge to Synthesize

Over the last decade, researchers across the disciplines have shown a growing interest in qualitative research synthesis. Especially notable in the practice disciplines (e.g., nursing, medicine, education), this new urge to synthesize is part of a larger movement to reduce the "information anxiety" (Harrison, 1996, p. 224) associated with the growth of empirical research and to facilitate better use of research findings (Cook, Mulrow, & Haynes, 1997) for the public health and welfare. Especially relevant to the surge of interest in qualitative research synthesis are the proliferation of qualitative studies over the last 20 years and the rise in the 1990s of evidence-based practice as a paradigm, methodology, and pedagogy for the practice disciplines. Qualitative research and evidence-based practice have become "growth industries" (Estabrooks, 1999, p. 274) that together are reshaping the conception of evidence and the practice of research synthesis.

ON THE CREST OF A WAVE

Qualitative research has been riding the "crest of a wave" (Morse, 1994) of popularity. Thousands of reports of qualitative studies have been published across the behavioral, social science, and practice disciplines. Especially notable is the upsurge in qualitative health research on such topics as: (a) the personal and cultural constructions of disease, prevention, treatment, and risk; (b) living with and managing the physical, psychological, and social effects of an array of diseases and their treatments; (c) decision making around and experiences with beginning- and end-of-life, and assistive and life-extending technological interventions; and (d) contextual (e.g., historical, cultural, political, discursive) factors favoring and impeding access to quality care, the promotion of good health, the

1

prevention of disease, and the reduction in health disparities. Reports of qualitative research now appear regularly, not only in exclusively qualitative research publication venues, but also in venues that once rejected qualitative studies as unscientific.

As qualitative research has become more prominent, so has concern about its value. Expressed in the now voluminous literature addressing what is variously referred to as the validity, quality, or rigor of qualitative research (e.g., Emden & Sandelowski, 1998, 1999; Maxwell, 1992; Seale, 1999), this concern has turned largely on the premise that qualitative research findings are not generalizable. Because they are derived from "small" and "non-representative" samples and "subjective" procedures, these findings are supposedly neither "reliable" nor "valid." Because they are putatively not generalizable, qualitative research findings can, therefore, not be used to resolve real-world problems. The irony here is that qualitative research is conducted in the real world—that is, in "natural" as opposed to the artificially controlled and/or manipulated conditions of quantitative research—yet it was viewed as producing findings not applicable in that world.

In response, proponents of qualitative research challenged prevailing assumptions and practices concerning validity and clarified the difference between the *nomothetic,* or formal, generalization that is the goal of quantitative research and the *idiographic,* or case-bound, generalization that is the goal of qualitative research. Nomothetic generalizations are drawn from statistically representative samples and applied to populations. Idiographic generalizations are drawn from and about informationally representative cases (Sandelowski, 1996a, 1997). Proponents also described the distinctive capacity of qualitative research for: (a) reaching facets of human experience out of the reach of quantitative methods; (b) developing, refining, and validating culturally sensitive instruments and participant-centered interventions; and for (c) augmenting the practical significance of, and even salvaging, quantitative research findings (Barroso & Sandelowski, 2001; Cohen, Kahn, & Steeves, 2002; Cohen & Saunders, 1996; Cox, 2003; Fountain & Griffiths, 1999; Gamel, Grypdonck, Hengeveld, & Davis, 2001; Gibson, Timlin, Curran, & Wattis, 2004; Kearney, 2001b; Mallinson, 2002; Miller, Druss, & Rohrbaugh, 2003; Morse, Hutchinson, & Penrod, 1998; Morse, Penrod, & Hupcey, 2000; Popay et al., 2003; Pope & Mays, 1995; Power, 1998; Sandelowski, 1996b, 1997, 2004; Swanson, Durham, & Albright, 1997; Thomas et al., 2004; Weinholtz, Kacer, & Rocklin, 1995).

Yet champions of qualitative research were also worried that qualitative inquiry was becoming a cottage industry, with researchers working in isolation from each other, producing "one-shot research" (Estabrooks,

Field, & Morse, 1994, p. 510) and, thereby, eternally reinventing the wheel. Early in the history of grounded theory, Glaser and Strauss (1971, p. 181) were concerned that the findings of individual studies would remain "little islands of knowledge" separated from one another and ultimately doomed never to be visited. Accordingly, despite its growing popularity, qualitative research appeared endangered by the failure to link individual studies. This failure was especially evident when compared to the surge of activity in quantitative research synthesis, especially the dramatic rise in popularity of quantitative meta-analysis, the constellation of statistical techniques developed to integrate quantitative research findings.

Qualitative research synthesis, thus, emerged in response to the proliferation but relative undervaluation and underutilization of the findings of qualitative studies. Proponents of qualitative inquiry hoped qualitative research synthesis (variously referred to as qualitative meta-analysis or qualitative metasynthesis) would take its rightful place alongside quantitative meta-analysis. Since its introduction in the mid-1970s, quantitative meta-analysis has come to be viewed as among the most significant methodologic advancements of the 20th century in bringing order to scientific inquiry, increasing the precision and power of research, and in enabling answers to questions not posed in and resolving controversies across primary quantitative studies (Alderson, Green, & Higgins, 2004). Proponents of a qualitative counterpart to quantitative meta-analysis hoped it would have as favorable an impact on qualitative research.

Quantitative meta-analysis also became central to evidence-based practice, the methodology that first emerged in the 1990s in the health disciplines to bridge the gap between research and practice. (Some critics of evidence-based practice contend that it is simply a new label for an old idea. For this and other critiques of evidence-based practice, see, e.g., Clarke, 1999; Estabrooks, 1999; Gupta, 2003; Hampton, 2002; Mykhalovskiy & Weir, 2004; Pellegrino, 2002; Timmermans & Berg, 2003; Traynor, 2002; Trinder, 2000). Now appearing in various guises across disciplines (e.g., as evidence-based health care, medicine, and nursing, and evidence-based education, social work, and librarianship; Trinder & Reynolds, 2000), evidence-based practice entails the systematic retrieval, evaluation, and synthesis of the best evidence available to serve as the basis for best practices (Sackett, Rosenberg, Gray, Haynes, & Richardson, 1996; Sackett, Straus, Richardson, Rosenberg, & Haynes, 2000). Therefore, the urge to synthesize qualitative research findings derives also from the desire to secure the place denied to qualitative research as a source of best evidence in the evidence-based practice process.

THE DEBATE OVER QUALITATIVE
RESEARCH SYNTHESIS

With the increasing turn to qualitative research synthesis has come controversy concerning how and even whether it is appropriate or feasible to synthesize qualitative research. At issue is whether qualitative research synthesis is an activity analogous to or wholly at odds with quantitative research synthesis. The questions yet to be fully answered are: Will qualitative research synthesis bring qualitative research to the center of inquiry and practice and, if so, at what cost to qualitative inquiry? Will mainstreaming qualitative research via research synthesis appreciate or depreciate the value of qualitative inquiry?

Appreciation and Legitimation

At one extreme end of the debate about qualitative research synthesis is the view that it enhances the value of qualitative research and the research synthesis enterprise, in general. Proponents of qualitative research synthesis conceive it as a way to bring qualitative research into the mainstream of inquiry that will, in turn, further legitimate the continued use of qualitative methods. Qualitative research is, in turn, viewed as essential to achieving the goal of evidence-based practice: namely to use the best evidence available as the foundation for practice without methodological prejudice.

Scholars eager to bring qualitative research and evidence-based practice together have called for the incorporation of qualitative studies in systematic reviews of research that had, heretofore, included only quantitative studies (Barbour, 2000; Dixon-Woods, Fitzpatrick, & Roberts, 2001; Green & Britten, 1998; Greenhalgh, 2002; Leys, 2003; Popay & Williams, 1998). The formation of the Cochrane Qualitative Research Methods Group, in association with the Cochrane Collaboration and Library (http://mysite.wanadoo-members.co.uk/Cochrane_Qual_Method/index.htm)—an icon of the movement toward evidence-based practice—is one outcome of the effort to align qualitative research with mainstream research synthesis efforts. Another outcome is the spate of literature that has appeared over the last decade advocating and describing methods to produce qualitative research syntheses (Beck, 2003; Britten et al., 2002; Campbell et al., 2003; Estabrooks, Field, & Morse, 1994; Finfgeld, 2003; Jensen & Allen, 1996; Kearney, 2001c; McCormick, Rodney, & Varcoe, 2003; Noblit & Hare, 1988; Paterson, Thorne, Canam, & Jillings, 2001; Sandelowski & Barroso, 2003a,b; Sandelowski, Docherty, & Emden, 1997; Schrieber, Crooks, & Stern, 1997; Sherwood, 1999), and reporting the results of reviews of research designated as qualitative research syntheses

(Arman & Rehnsfeldt, 2003; Barroso & Powell-Cope, 2000; Beck, 2001, 2002a,b; Bowers, 2002; Burke, Kauffmann, Costello, Wiskin, & Harrison, 1998; Carroll, 2004; Clemmens, 2003; Finfgeld, 1999, 2000; Jensen & Allen, 1994; Kearney, 1998b, 2001a; Kearney & O'Sullivan, 2003; Kennedy, Rousseau, & Low, 2003; McNaughton, 2000; Meadows-Oliver, 2003; Nelson, 2002, 2003; Paterson, 2001; Paterson, Thorne, & Dewis, 1998; Sherwood, 1997). In these works, qualitative research synthesis is an opportunity to enhance the "utilization value" (Smaling, 2003, pp. 20–21) and "power" (Kearney, 1998a, p. 182) of qualitative research findings. *Power* here refers, not to the ability to generalize from representative samples to populations (as in the formal generalization sought in quantitative research), but rather to the ability to generalize from and about cases across a range of cases (or the idiographic generalization characterizing qualitative research; Sandelowski, 1996a). Schofield (1990) viewed qualitative research syntheses as cross-case generalizations created from the case-bound generalizations in individual studies. Idiographic knowledge, or knowledge of the particular, is viewed as especially critical in the practice disciplines, where knowledge must always be fitted to the individual case and the particular circumstance (Hunter, 1991). As champions of qualitative research have argued, the development of valid and culturally sensitive instruments and effective participant-centered interventions ultimately depends on the kind of idiographic knowledge only qualitative inquiry yields.

Depreciation and Cooptation

At the other extreme end of the debate is the view that even the thought of synthesizing qualitative research findings violates the assumptions and imperatives of qualitative research. Qualitative research synthesis is here seen as an effort to mainstream qualitative inquiry that will ultimately end in its cooptation. Practices such as qualitative inquiry are commandeered or appropriated to reduce the threat they pose to prevailing practices. In the process of cooptation, these practices are assimilated and, thereby, weakened and even erased as they are brought into conformity with the very practices they were meant to subvert. Indeed, after successful cooptation, the very problems that the threatening idea was intended to resolve are reproduced. Evidence-based practice is seen as an effort to minimize the impact of qualitative research by enforcing models of valid science and good scholarship that are at odds with it and, thereby, to neutralize its critique of mainstream research (Lincoln, 2005). The realist stance of evidence-based practice is seen to conflict with the relativist stance of postmodern inquiry, which has had such a profound influence on qualitative research. Whereas evidence-based practice emphasizes generalizing, averaging, and the resolution of contradictions, qualitative research—especially under the influence of postmodern inquiry—emphasizes the impossibility and even the fallacy of generalizing, difference and variation, and the representation of contradictions (Clarke, 2005). Metaphorically, while evidence-based practice emphasizes the pointed end of a funnel (i.e., an end-product, a result, coming to a point), qualitative research emphasizes the open end of a funnel (i.e., the practice of inquiry and the implausibility of any one point).

Accordingly, despite the apparent rapprochement between qualitative research and evidence-based practice, a central issue to those more wary of the growing popularity of qualitative research synthesis is whether the evidence-based practice paradigm—and the quantitatively informed systematic reviews of research at its center—is compatible with the imperatives of qualitative research, especially a qualitative research increasingly under the influence of postmodern ideas. Most systematic reviews of research have been based largely on hierarchical ratings of evidence (DeBourgh, 2001, p. 463) in which the randomized controlled trial is viewed as offering the best evidence and qualitative research is viewed as offering the worst or no evidence at all (Lohr & Carey, 1999; West et al., 2002). Advocates of qualitative research have argued that by treating the randomized controlled trial as the gold standard in inquiry and, thereby, depreciating or frankly excluding qualitative research from consideration as evidence, evidence-based practice reinforces well-worn prejudices against qualitative research (Evans, 2003; McKenna, Cutliffe, & McKenna, 1999; Mitchell, 1999). Advocates of qualitative research and critics of the evidence-based practice movement have further contended that the evidence hierarchies driving evidence-based practice reify the very idea of evidence. Evidence is not a stable commodity that is obtained by adhering to standardized procedure, but rather an evolving entity; what is deemed to be evidence is always theoretically informed, historically situated, socially constructed, and even politically motivated (Eisner, 1991; Fawcett, Watson, Neuman, Walker, & Fitzpatrick, 2001; Forbes et al., 1999; Hampton, 2002; Madjar & Walton, 2001; Miller & Fredericks, 2003; Ray & Mayan, 2001; Upshur, 2001a,b; Zarkovich & Upshur, 2002).

Advocates of qualitative research and critics of evidence-based practice view the emphasis on standardization of and conformity to procedure that characterizes the discussion and implementation of evidence-based practice as conflicting with the antistandardization and anticonformity impulses of qualitative research. Evidence-based practice is here deemed to constitute yet another disciplinary technology (Walker, 2003) that only serves to enforce the conformity of qualitative inquiry to standards for quantitative inquiry, to reinforce false and invidious distinctions between qualitative and quantitative research and, thereby, to reproduce the very problems it was intended to solve. Most notable among these problems are the failure to use all of the best evidence available for practice, conduct judicious appraisals of disparate forms of evidence, and develop the critical consciousness (Berkwits, 1998) that offset the dogmatism characterizing many efforts to promote evidence-based practice (Traynor, 1999).

Can You Sum Up a Poem?

In addition to the perceived philosophical incompatibility between evidence-based practice and qualitative research, advocates of qualitative research contend that the very nature of qualitative research makes it resistant to synthesis. Efforts to synthesize qualitative findings seem to undermine the "function and provenance" of cases (Davis, 1991, p. 12) and to sacrifice the vitality, viscerality, and vicariousness of the human experiences represented in the original studies. The very emphasis in qualitative research on the complexities and contradictions of "N=1 experiences" (Eisner, 1991, p. 197) arguably precludes efforts to aggregate them in ways analogous to quantitative research synthesis. In short, qualitative research is viewed to be as resistant to synthesis as are poems.

Even assuming that qualitative research findings can and ought to be synthesized, the sheer diversity in the implementation and reporting of qualitative research poses challenges to synthesis. As champions of qualitative inquiry have recurrently argued, a hallmark of qualitative research is "variability," not "standardization" (Popay, Rogers, & Williams, 1998, p. 346). The highly diverse commitments to and training in qualitative research within and across disciplines have resulted in highly disparate methods for conducting qualitative inquiry. In addition, a commonplace in qualitative research is that "one narrative size does not fit all" (Tierney, 1995, p. 389) in the reporting of qualitative studies, with write-ups ranging from the conventional scientific experimental/APA style of reporting to deliberately anti-experimental and artistic ventures in representation. (Reporting styles are addressed in more detail in chapters 4 and 9.) Accordingly, highly disparate activities are designated as qualitative inquiry, highly disparate methodological approaches are designated as the same method (e.g., grounded theory, phenomenology), and the identification of findings to synthesize in qualitative research reports is itself often a daunting task (Sandelowski & Barroso, 2002).

Qualitative research proponents concerned about the impact of the urge to synthesize on qualitative research also caution against reliance on quantitative meta-analysis as the model for the development and implementation of qualitative research synthesis. Calling for synthesis methods distinctive to qualitative inquiry (Barbour & Barbour, 2003; Jones, 2004;

Sandelowski, Docherty, & Emden, 1997), proponents of qualitative research have yet to reach consensus on: (a) terminology (e.g., qualitative meta-analysis [or meta analysis], meta-synthesis [or metasynthesis], metadata-analysis); (b) whether to match integration methods to the methods named in the primary studies (i.e., using grounded theory to synthesize studies designated as grounded theory); (c) whether to retrieve all of the research reports in a targeted domain or only a purposeful sample of them; (d) what the goal(s) of qualitative research synthesis should be (e.g., topical review, aggregation, integration, interpretive comparison, critique); (e) how to conduct qualitative research syntheses; and (f) whether to advance one or multiple interpretations of studies (Booth, 2001; Doyle, 2003; Evans & Pearson, 2001; Jones, 2004; Noblit & Hare, 1988; Thorne, Jensen, Kearney, Noblit, & Sandelowski, 2004).

Further complicating the qualitative research enterprise is its very methodological appeal and cachet. Because qualitative research synthesis—like qualitative research—is riding the crest of a wave of popularity, more entities are being designated as qualitative research syntheses that are nothing more than conventional impressionistic reviews of the literature or inventories of the topics and methods covered in a targeted body of research. These professed syntheses of qualitative research findings have become increasingly attractive to persons seeking to bypass the challenges of human subjects research, who see qualitative research as an entrée into research less challenging than quantitative research (Thorne et al., 2004), and who seek the "epistemological credibility" (Thorne, Kirkham, & MacDonald-Emes, 1997, p. 170) and "rhetorical advantages" (Seale, 2002, p. 659) of naming their work *qualitative research synthesis*. This form of conceptual drift, whereby a concept (i.e., qualitative research synthesis) comes to include an increasing number of disparate entities, elides the differences between true qualitative research synthesis and the kind of unsystematic review of the literature proponents of quantitative meta-analysis designate as "qualitative" or "narrative" and disparage as too subjective and unsystematic. Conceptual drift reinforces the view of the *systematic* and *qualitative* review of qualitative research findings as an oxymoron, the practice of designating any nonstatistical treatment of literature as *qualitative,* and the tendency to confuse the mere presentation of data with interpretation (see chapter 5). For example, merely naming—and counting the number of studies addressing—the topics covered in a selected group of studies is not the same as systematically integrating the results of those studies. The qualitative research synthesis enterprise thus remains conflated with other activities seen as lacking in depth and scientific credibility. More ominously, qualitative research synthesis is in danger of meaning nothing because it means too much.

QUALITATIVE RESEARCH SYNTHESIS
AS A CONTESTED SITE

We created this *Handbook* mindful of the historical context for qualitative research synthesis, and of the competing interpretations of qualitative research synthesis and the reasons for the turn and resistance to it. Whereas some members of the qualitative research community see this turn as advancing qualitative research, others view it as dangerous to it—even as a manifestation of a "backlash" (Denzin & Lincoln, 2005, p. 3) against it. While qualitative research synthesis is being pulled hard on the one side toward the generalizing imperatives of evidence-based practice, it is also being pulled hard on the other side toward the anti-generalizing impulses of postmodern inquiry. (See Figure 1.1.) But the very existence of this book indicates our belief that qualitative research synthesis is a possible and worthy activity precisely because of—and when conducted with acknowledgment of—these opposing strains.

We are also not naive to the challenges and even dangers involved in articulating methods, not the least of which is being seen to be prescribing or legislating only one way of doing things and, thereby, reinforcing a preoccupation with method over substance. We know that methods have multiple existences as: (a) ways of gaining access to something heretofore unknown; (b) interventions into or "interference(s)" (Mol, 2002, p. 155) with the unknown (by virtue of the activities engaged in to secure that access); and (c) themselves unknowns, when methods are treated as the objects (as opposed to means) of inquiry. The methods we feature in the chapters that follow reflect, in ways that we hope preserve

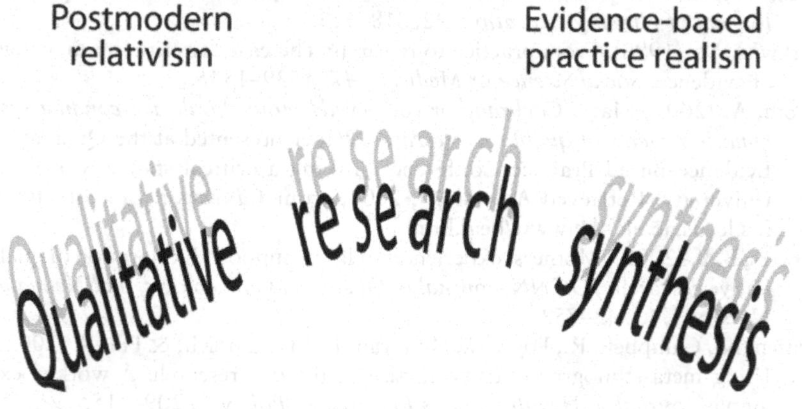

Postmodern
relativism

Evidence-based
practice realism

Qualitative research synthesis

FIGURE 1.1 Opposing forces on qualitative research synthesis.

the integrity and enhance the utility of qualitative research for practice, our understanding of, and solutions for, the challenges qualitative research synthesis—as method and subject matter—poses.

REFERENCES

Alderson, P., Green, S., & Higgins, J.P.T. (Eds.). (2004, March). *Cochrane reviewers' handbook 4.2.2* [updated quarterly]. In The Cochrane Library, Issue 1, 2004. Chichester, UK: John Wiley & Sons, Ltd. Retrieved May 11, 2004, from http://www.cochrane.org/ resources/handbook/hbook.htm

Arman, M., & Rehnsfeldt, A. (2003). The hidden suffering among breast cancer patients: A qualitative metasynthesis. *Qualitative Health Research, 13,* 510–527.

Barbour, R. S. (2000). The role of qualitative research in broadening the "evidence base" for clinical practice. *Journal of Evaluation in Clinical Practice, 6,* 155–163.

Barbour, R. S., & Barbour, M. (2003). Evaluating and synthesizing qualitative research: The need to develop a distinctive approach. *Journal of Evaluation in Clinical Practice, 9,* 179–186.

Barroso, J., & Powell-Cope, G. M. (2000). Metasynthesis of qualitative research on living with HIV infection. *Qualitative Health Research, 10,* 340–353.

Barroso, J., & Sandelowski, M. (2001). In the field with the Beck Depression Inventory. *Qualitative Health Research, 11,* 491–504.

Beck, C. T. (2001). Caring within nursing education: A metasynthesis. *Journal of Nursing Education, 40,* 101–109.

Beck, C. T. (2002a). Mothering multiples: A meta-synthesis of qualitative research. *MCN: American Journal of Maternal Child Nursing, 27,* 214–221.

Beck, C. T. (2002b). Postpartum depression: A metasynthesis. *Qualitative Health Research, 12,* 453–472.

Beck, C. T. (2003). Seeing the forest for the trees: A qualitative synthesis project. *Journal of Nursing Education, 42,* 318–323.

Berkwits, M. (1998). From practice to research: The case for criticism in an age of evidence. *Social Science & Medicine, 47,* 1539–1545.

Booth, A. (2001, May). *Cochrane or cock-eyed? How should we conduct systematic reviews of qualitative research?* Paper presented at the Qualitative Evidence-Based Practice Conference: Taking a critical stance, Coventry University. Retrieved August 25, 2004, from *Education-Line* at http://brs.leeds.ac.uk/~beiwww/beid.html

Bowers, B. B. (2002). Mothers' experiences of labor support: Exploration of qualitative research. *JOGNN: Journal of Obstetric, Gynecologic, and Neonatal Nursing, 31,* 742–752.

Britten, N., Campbell, R., Pope, C., Donovan, J., Morgan, M., & Pill, R. (2002). Using meta-ethnography to synthesize qualitative research: A worked example. *Journal of Health Services Research & Policy, 7,* 209–215.

Burke, S. O., Kauffmann, E., Costello, E., Wiskin, N., & Harrison, M. B. (1998).

Stressors in families with a child with a chronic condition: An analysis of qualitative studies and a framework. *Canadian Journal of Nursing Research, 30(1),* 71–95.

Campbell, R., Pound, P., Pope, C., Britten, N., Pill, R., Morgan, M., et al. (2003). Evaluating meta-ethnography: A synthesis of qualitative research on lay experiences of diabetes and diabetes care. *Social Science & Medicine, 56,* 671–684.

Carroll, S. M. (2004). Nonvocal ventilated patients' perceptions of being understood. *Western Journal of Nursing Research, 26,* 85–103.

Clarke, A. E. (2005). *Situational analysis: Grounded theory after the postmodern turn.* Thousand Oaks, CA: Sage.

Clarke, J. B. (1999). Evidence-based practice: A retrograde step? The importance of pluralism in evidence generation for the practice of health care. *Journal of Clinical Nursing, 8,* 89–94.

Clemmens, D. (2003). Adolescent motherhood: A meta-synthesis of qualitative studies. *MCN: American Journal of Maternal Child Nursing, 28,* 93–99.

Cohen, M. Z., Kahn, D. L., & Steeves, R. H. (2002). Making use of qualitative research. *Western Journal of Nursing Research, 24,* 454–471.

Cohen, M. Z., & Saunders, J. M. (1996). Using qualitative research in advanced practice. *Advanced Nursing Practice Quarterly, 2(3),* 8–13.

Cook, D. J., Mulrow, C. D., & Haynes, R. B. (1997). Systematic reviews: Synthesis of best evidence for clinical decisions. *Annals of Internal Medicine, 126,* 376–380.

Cox, K. (2003). Assessing the quality of life of patients in phase I and phase II anti-cancer drug trials: Interviews versus questionnaires. *Social Science & Medicine, 56,* 921–934.

Davis, D. S. (1991). Rich cases: The ethics of thick description. *Hastings Center Report, 21(4),* 12–17.

DeBourgh, G. A. (2001). Evidence-based practice: Fad or functional paradigm? *AACN Clinical Issues, 12,* 463–467.

Denzin, N. K., & Lincoln, Y. S. (2005). Introduction: The discipline and practice of qualitative research. In N. K. Denzin & Y. S. Lincoln (Eds.), *The Sage handbook of qualitative research* (3rd ed., pp. 1–32). Thousand Oaks, CA: Sage.

Dixon-Woods, M., Fitzpatrick, R., & Roberts, K. (2001). Including qualitative research in systematic reviews: Opportunities and problems. *Journal of Evaluation in Clinical Practice, 7,* 125–133.

Doyle, L. H. (2003). Synthesis through meta-ethnography: Paradoxes, enhancements, and possibilities. *Qualitative Research, 3,* 321–345.

Eisner, E. W. (1991). *The enlightened eye: Qualitative inquiry and the enhancement of educational practice.* New York: Macmillan.

Emden, C., & Sandelowski, M. (1998). The good, the bad, and the relative, part 1: Conceptions of goodness in qualitative research. *International Journal of Nursing Practice, 4,* 206–212.

Emden, C., & Sandelowski, M. (1999). The good, the bad, and the relative, part 2: Goodness and the criterion problem in qualitative research. *International Journal of Nursing Practice, 5,* 2–7.

Estabrooks, C. A. (1999). Will evidence-based nursing practice make practice perfect? *Canadian Journal of Nursing Research, 30,* 273–294.

Estabrooks, C. A., Field, P. A., & Morse, J. M. (1994). Aggregating qualitative findings: An approach to theory development. *Qualitative Health Research, 4,* 503–511.

Evans, D. (2003). Hierarchy of evidence: A framework for ranking evidence evaluating health care interventions. *Journal of Clinical Nursing, 12,* 77–84.

Evans, D., & Pearson, A. (2001). Systematic reviews of qualitative research. *Clinical Effectiveness in Nursing, 5,* 111-119 (with commentaries and author response).

Fawcett, J., Watson, J., Neuman, B., Walker, P. H., & Fitzpatrick, J. J. (2001). On nursing theories and evidence. *Journal of Nursing Scholarship, 33,* 115–119.

Finfgeld, D. L. (1999). Courage as a process of pushing beyond the struggle. *Qualitative Health Research, 9,* 803–814.

Finfgeld, D. L. (2000). Self-resolution of drug and alcohol problems: A synthesis of qualitative findings. *Journal of Addictions Nursing, 12,* 65–72.

Finfgeld, D. L. (2003). Metasynthesis: The state of the art—so far. *Qualitative Health Research, 13,* 893–904.

Forbes, D. A., King, K. M., Kushner, K. E., Letourneau, N. L., Myrick, A. F., & Profetto-McGrath, J. (1999). Warrantable evidence in nursing science. *Journal of Advanced Nursing, 29,* 373–379.

Fountain, J., & Griffiths, P. (1999). Synthesis of qualitative research on drug use in the European Union: Report on an EMCDDA Project. *European Addiction Research, 5,* 4–20.

Gamel, C., Grypdonck, M., Hengeveld, M., & Davis, B. (2001). A method to develop a nursing intervention: The contribution of qualitative studies to the process. *Journal of Advanced Nursing, 33,* 806–819.

Gibson, G., Timlin, A., Curran, S., & Wattis, J. (2004). The scope for qualitative methods in research and clinical trials in dementia. *Age and Ageing, 33,* 422–426.

Glaser, B. G., & Strauss, A. L. (1971). *Status passage.* Chicago: Aldine.

Green, J., & Britten, N. (1998). Qualitative research and evidence based medicine. *British Medical Journal, 316,* 1230–1232.

Greenhalgh, T. (2002). Integrating qualitative research into evidence based practice. *Endocrinology and Metabolism Clinics of North America, 31,* 583–601.

Gupta, M. (2003). A critical appraisal of evidence-based medicine: Some ethical considerations. *Journal of Evaluation in Clinical Practice, 9,* 111–121.

Hampton, J. R. (2002). Evidence-based medicine, opinion-based medicine, and real-world medicine. *Perspectives in Biology and Medicine, 45,* 549-568.

Harrison, L. L. (1996). Pulling it all together: The importance of integrative research reviews and meta-analyses in nursing (Editorial). *Journal of Advanced Nursing, 24,* 224–225.

Hunter, K. M. (1991). *Doctor's stories: The narrative structure of medical knowledge.* Princeton, NJ: Princeton University Press.

Jensen, L. A., & Allen, M. N. (1994). A synthesis of qualitative research on wellness-illness. *Qualitative Health Research, 4,* 349–369.

Jensen, L. A., & Allen, M. N. (1996). Meta-synthesis of qualitative findings. *Qualitative Health Research, 6,* 553–560.

Jones, K. (2004). Mission drift in qualitative research, or moving toward a systematic review of qualitative studies, moving back to a more systematic narrative review. *The Qualitative Report, 9(1),* 95–112. Retrieved August 29, 2004, from www.nova.edu/ssss/ QR/QR9-1/jones.pdf

Kearney, M. H. (1998a). Ready-to-wear: Discovering grounded formal theory. *Research in Nursing & Health, 21,* 179–186.

Kearney, M. H. (1998b). Truthful self-nurturing: A grounded formal theory of women's addiction recovery. *Qualitative Health Research, 8,* 495–512.

Kearney, M. H. (2001a). Enduring love: A grounded formal theory of women's experience of domestic violence. *Research in Nursing & Health, 24,* 270–282.

Kearney, M. H. (2001b). Levels and applications of qualitative research evidence. *Research in Nursing & Health, 24,* 145–153.

Kearney, M. H. (2001c). New directions in grounded formal theory. In R. Schreiber & P. N. Stern (Eds.), *Using grounded theory in nursing* (pp. 227–246). New York: Springer Publishing.

Kearney, M. H., & O'Sullivan, J. (2003). Identity shifts as turning points in health behavior change. *Western Journal of Nursing Research, 25,* 134–152.

Kennedy, H. P., Rousseau, A. L., & Low, L. K. (2003). An exploratory metasynthesis of midwifery practice in the United States. *Midwifery, 19,* 203–214.

Leys, M. (2003). Health care policy: Qualitative evidence and health technology assessment. *Health Policy, 65,* 217–226.

Lincoln, Y. S. (2005). Institutional review boards and methodological conservatism: The challenge to and from phenomenological paradigms. In N. K. Denzin & Y. S. Lincoln (Eds.), *The Sage handbook of qualitative research* (3rd ed., pp. 165–181). Thousand Oaks, CA: Sage.

Lohr, K. N., & Carey, T. S. (1999). Assessing "best evidence": Issues in grading the quality of studies for systematic reviews. *Joint Commission Journal on Quality Improvement, 25,* 470–479.

Madjar, I., & Walton, J. A. (2001). What is problematic about evidence? In J. M. Morse, J. M. Swanson, & A. J. Kuzel (Eds.), *The nature of qualitative evidence* (pp. 28–45). Thousand Oaks, CA: Sage.

Mallinson, S. (2002). Listening to respondents: A qualitative assessment of the Short-Form 36 Health Status Questionnaire. *Social Science & Medicine, 54,* 11–21.

Maxwell, J. A. (1992). Understanding and validity in qualitative research. *Harvard Educational Review, 62,* 279–300.

McCormick, J., Rodney, P., & Varcoe, C. (2003). Reinterpretations across studies: An approach to meta-analysis. *Qualitative Health Research, 13,* 933–944.

McKenna, H., Cutliffe, J., & McKenna, P. (1999). Evidence-based practice: Demolishing some myths. *Nursing Standard, 14,* 39–42.

McNaughton, D. B. (2000). A synthesis of qualitative home visiting research. *Public Health Nursing, 17,* 405–414.

Meadows-Oliver, M. (2003). Mothering in public: A meta-synthesis of homeless women with children living in shelters. *JSPN, Journal for Specialists in Pediatric Nursing, 8*, 130–136.

Miller, C. L., Druss, B. G., & Rohrbaugh, R. M. (2003). Using qualitative methods to distill the active ingredients of a multifaceted intervention. *Psychiatric Services, 54*, 568–571.

Miller, S., & Fredericks, M. (2003). The nature of "evidence" in qualitative research methods. *International Journal of Qualitative Methods, 2(1)*. Article 4. Retrieved September 22, 2003, from http://www.ualberta.ca/~iiqm/backissues/2_1/html/miller.html

Mitchell, G. J. (1999). Evidence-based practice: Critique and alternative view. *Nursing Science Quarterly, 12*, 30–35.

Mol, A. (2002). *The body multiple: Ontology in medical practice.* Durham, NC: Duke University Press.

Morse, J. M. (1994). On the crest of a wave? (Editorial). *Qualitative Health Research, 4*, 139–141.

Morse, J. M., Hutchinson, S. A., & Penrod, J. (1998). From theory to practice: The development of assessment guides from qualitatively derived theory. *Qualitative Health Research, 8*, 329–340.

Morse, J. M., Penrod, J., & Hupcey, J. E. (2000). Qualitative outcome analysis: Evaluating nursing interventions for complex clinical phenomena. *Journal of Nursing Scholarship, 32*, 125–130.

Mykhalovskiy, E., & Weir, L. (2004). The problem of evidence-based medicine: Directions for social science. *Social Science & Medicine, 59*, 1059–1069.

Nelson, A. M. (2002). A metasynthesis: Mothering other-than-normal children. *Qualitative Health Research, 12*, 515–530.

Nelson, A. M. (2003). Transition to motherhood. *JOGNN: Journal of Obstetric, Gynecologic, and Neonatal Nursing, 32*, 465–477.

Noblit, G. W., & Hare, R. D. (1988). *Meta-ethnography: Synthesizing qualitative studies.* Newbury Park, CA: Sage.

Paterson, B. L. (2001). The shifting perspectives model of chronic illness. *Journal of Nursing Scholarship, 33*, 21–26.

Paterson, B. L., Thorne, S. E., Canam, C., & Jillings, C. (2001). *Meta-study of qualitative health research: A practical guide to meta-analysis and meta-synthesis.* Thousand Oaks, CA: Sage.

Paterson, B. L., Thorne, S., & Dewis, M. (1998). Adapting to and managing diabetes. *Image: Journal of Nursing Scholarship, 30*, 57–62.

Pellegrino, E. D. (2002). Medical evidence and virtue ethics: A commentary on Zarkovich and Upshur. *Theoretical Medicine, 23*, 397–402.

Popay, J., Bennett, S., Thomas, C., Williams, G., Gatrell, A., & Bostock, L. (2003). Beyond "beer, fags, egg and chips"? Exploring lay understandings of social inequalities in health. *Sociology of Health & Illness, 25*, 1–23.

Popay, J., Rogers, A., & Williams, G. (1998). Rationale and standards for the systematic review of qualitative literature in health services research. *Qualitative Health Research, 8*, 341–351.

Popay, J., & Williams, G. (1998). Qualitative research and evidence-based health care. *Journal of the Royal Society of Medicine, 91 (Suppl. 35)*, 32–37.

Pope, C., & Mays, N. (1995). Reaching the parts other methods cannot reach: An introduction to qualitative methods in health and health services research. *British Medical Journal, 311,* 42–45.

Power, R. (1998). The role of qualitative research in HIV/AIDS. *AIDS, 12,* 687–695.

Ray, L. D., & Mayan, M. (2001). Who decides what counts as evidence? In J. M. Morse, J. M. Swanson, & A. J. Kuzel (Eds.), *The nature of qualitative evidence* (pp. 50–73). Thousand Oaks, CA: Sage.

Sackett, D. L., Rosenberg, W. M., Gray, J. A., Haynes, R. B., & Richardson, W. S. (1996). Evidence based medicine: What it is and what it isn't. *British Medical Journal, 312(7023),* 71–72.

Sackett, D. L.. Straus, S. E., Richardson, W. S., Rosenberg, W., & Haynes, R. B. (2000). *Evidence-based medicine: How to practice and teach EBM.* Edinburgh: Churchill Livingstone.

Sandelowski, M. (1996a). One is the liveliest number: The case orientation of qualitative research. *Research in Nursing & Health, 19,* 525–529.

Sandelowski, M. (1996b). Using qualitative methods in intervention studies. *Research in Nursing & Health, 19,* 359–364.

Sandelowski, M. (1997). "To be of use": Enhancing the utility of qualitative research. *Nursing Outlook, 45,* 125–132.

Sandelowski, M. (2004). Using qualitative research. *Qualitative Health Research, 14,* 1366–1386.

Sandelowski, M., & Barroso, J. (2002). Finding the findings in qualitative studies. *Journal of Nursing Scholarship, 34,* 213–219.

Sandelowski, M., & Barroso, J. (2003a). Creating metasummaries of qualitative findings. *Nursing Research, 52,* 226–233.

Sandelowski, M., & Barroso, J. (2003b). Toward a metasynthesis of qualitative findings on motherhood in HIV-positive women. *Research in Nursing & Health, 26,* 153–170.

Sandelowski, M., Docherty, S., & Emden, C. (1997). Qualitative metasynthesis: Issues and techniques. *Research in Nursing & Health, 20,* 365–371.

Schofield, J. W. (1990). Increasing the generalizability of qualitative research. In E. W. Eisner & A. Peshkin (Eds.), *Qualitative inquiry in education: The continuing debate* (pp. 201–232). New York: Teachers College Press.

Schreiber, R., Crooks, D., & Stern, P. N. (1997). Qualitative meta-analysis. In J. M. Morse (Ed.), *Completing a qualitative project* (pp. 311–326). Thousand Oaks, CA: Sage.

Seale, C. (1999). *The quality of qualitative research.* London: Sage.

Seale, C. F. (2002). Computer-assisted analysis of qualitative interview data. In J. F. Gubrium & J. A. Holstein (Eds.), *Handbook of interview research: Context & method* (pp. 651–670). Thousand Oaks, CA: Sage.

Sherwood, G. D. (1997). Metasynthesis of qualitative analyses of caring: Defining a therapeutic model of nursing. *Advanced Practice Nursing Quarterly, 3,* 32–42.

Sherwood, G. (1999). Meta-synthesis: Merging qualitative studies to develop nursing knowledge. *International Journal of Human Caring, 3,* 37–42.

Smaling, A. (2003). Inductive, analogical, and communicative generalization. *International Journal of Qualitative Methods, 2(1)*. Article 5. Retrieved September 22, 2003, from http://www.ualberta.ca/~iiqm/backissues/2_1/html/smaling.html

Swanson, J. M., Durham, R. F., & Albright, J. (1997). Clinical utilization/application of qualitative research. In J. M. Morse (Ed.), *Completing a qualitative project* (pp. 253–281). Thousand Oaks, CA: Sage.

Thomas, J., Harden, A., Oakley, A., Oliver, S., Sutcliffe, K., Rees, R., et al. (2004). Integrating qualitative research with trials in systematic reviews. *British Medical Journal, 328*, 1010–1012.

Thorne, S., Jensen, L., Kearney, M. H., Noblit, G., & Sandelowski, M. (2004). Qualitative meta-synthesis: Reflections on methodological orientation and ideological agenda. *Qualitative Health Research, 14*, 1342–1365.

Thorne, S., Kirkham, S. R., & MacDonald-Emes, J. (1997). Interpretive description: A noncategorical qualitative alternative for developing nursing knowledge. *Research in Nursing & Health, 20*, 169–177.

Tierney, W. G. (1995). (Re)Presentation and voice. *Qualitative Inquiry, 1*, 379–390.

Timmermans, S., & Berg, M. (2003). *The gold standard: The challenge of evidence-based medicine and standardization in health care.* Philadelphia: Temple University Press.

Traynor, M. (1999). The problem of dissemination: Evidence and ideology. *Nursing Inquiry, 6*, 187–197.

Traynor, M. (2002). The oil crisis, risk and evidence-based practice. *Nursing Inquiry, 9*, 162–169.

Trinder, L. (2000). A critical appraisal of evidence-based practice. In L. Trinder & S. Reynolds (Eds.), *Evidence-based practice: A critical appraisal* (pp. 212–241). Oxford, UK: Blackwell Science.

Trinder, L., & Reynolds, S. (Eds.). (2000). *Evidence-based practice: A critical appraisal.* Oxford, UK: Blackwell Science.

Upshur, R. E. G. (2001a). The ethics of alpha: Reflections on statistics, evidence and values in medicine. *Theoretical Medicine, 22*, 565–576.

Upshur, R. E. G. (2001b). The status of qualitative research as evidence. In J. M. Morse, J. M. Swanson, & A. J. Kuzel (Eds.), *The nature of qualitative evidence* (pp. 5–26). Thousand Oaks, CA: Sage.

Walker, K. (2003). Why evidence-based practice now? A polemic. *Nursing Inquiry, 10*, 145–155.

Weinholtz, D. Kacer, B., & Rocklin, T. (1995). Salvaging quantitative research with qualitative data. *Qualitative Health Research, 5*, 388–397.

West, S., King, V., Carey, T. S., Lohr, K. N., McKoy, N., Sutton, S. F., et al. (2002, April). *Systems to rate the strength of scientific evidence.* Evidence Report/Technology Assessment No. 47, AHRQ Pub. No. 02-E016. Rockville, MD: Agency for Healthcare Research and Quality.

Zarkovich, E., & Upshur, R. E. G. (2002). The virtues of evidence. *Theoretical Medicine, 23*, 403–412.

CHAPTER TWO

Conceiving the Qualitative Research Synthesis Study

To begin your project, you must have a clear sense of what qualitative research synthesis is as opposed to other kinds of qualitative syntheses and reviews of the literature. You must also formulate a research purpose that addresses a clearly defined and significant research problem, consider the resources your project will require, and accommodate it to the resources available to you.

QUALITATIVE RESEARCH SYNTHESIS

Qualitative research synthesis refers to a process and product of scientific inquiry aimed at systematically reviewing and formally integrating the findings in reports of completed qualitative studies. Qualitative research synthesis projects encompass a family of methodological approaches. Methods are accommodated to the reports that comprise the body of empirical literature in a field of study and to the research purpose for the synthesis project. Accordingly, method enters qualitative research synthesis studies by way of reviewers' purposes and their appraisal of the findings themselves, not by way of the method claims in individual reports, or reviewers' allegiance to any one method or to any one approach toward executing that method.

In this book, we feature two large categories of qualitative research synthesis (see chapters 6 and 7). *Qualitative metasummary* is a quantitatively oriented aggregation of qualitative research findings that are themselves topical or thematic summaries or surveys of data. Metasummaries are integrations that approximate the sum of findings across reports in a target domain of research. They address the manifest content in findings, reflect a view of language as a neutral vehicle of communication, and show a quantitative logic: to discern the frequency of each finding, and to find in higher frequency findings the evidence of replication foundational to validity in quantitative research and to the claim of having discovered a pattern or theme in qualitative research (Sandelowski, 2001). Qualitative metasummaries may be an end in themselves, or they may serve as an empirical foundation for, or bridge to, qualitative metasynthesis, preparing survey findings for qualitative metasynthesis and optimizing the validity of the syntheses produced.

Qualitative metasynthesis is an interpretive integration of qualitative findings that are themselves interpretive syntheses of data, including the phenomenologies, ethnographies, grounded theories, and other coherent descriptions or explanations of phenomena, events, or cases that are the hallmark findings of qualitative research. Metasyntheses are integrations that are more than the sum of parts in that they offer novel interpretations of findings that are the result of interpretive transformations far removed from these findings as given in research reports. Although faithful to the findings in each report, these interpretations will not be found in any one research report, but rather comprise an integration derived from taking all of the reports in a sample as a whole. Metasyntheses offer a fully integrated description or explanation of a target event or experience, instead of a summary view of unlinked features of that event or experience. Such interpretive integrations require researchers to piece the individual syntheses constituting the findings in individual primary research reports together to craft one or more metasyntheses. In contrast to qualitative metasummary, which emphasizes reportage and a surface penetration of research findings, qualitative metasynthesis emphasizes the more penetrating interpretive acts of reading into and between the lines and over-reading (Poirier & Ayres, 1997). In qualitative metasyntheses, language is viewed as a structure or artifact of culture that must itself be interpreted. Their validity does not reside in a replication logic, but rather in an interpretive logic, whereby findings are reframed, and in the craftsmanship exhibited in the final product.

QUALITATIVE RESEARCH SYNTHESIS
VERSUS OTHER ENTITIES

Although it has features that overlap with other forms of inquiry, qualitative research synthesis is different from: (a) other reviews of the literature (i.e., the background review, the narrative overview of a research domain); (b) other research syntheses (i.e., quantitative or qualitative syntheses of quantitative research findings); (c) secondary analysis; (d) other syntheses found in qualitative inquiry (i.e., constituting the findings within primary studies, constituting an integration or reinterpretation of findings across a program of research); and from (e) other studies of studies (i.e., metastudy). (See Tables 2.1 and 2.2.)

In Contrast to the Background Review

In contrast to the background review of literature that is the prelude to a specific study, qualitative research synthesis—by itself—constitutes a form of scientific inquiry. Those who conduct qualitative research synthesis studies have the same obligations to execute these studies in as systematic and justifiable a manner as researchers conducting studies with human subjects. For example, those who conduct qualitative research synthesis studies have the same obligation to detail and defend the inclusion and exclusion criteria—and to summarize the relevant features—of their samples as researchers conducting studies with human subjects. But the samples in research synthesis studies are composed of research reports, not human subjects. The narrative background review of the literature that typically precedes the proposal or report of a primary study is designed to link selected studies in one or more fields in a chain of reasoning (Doyle, 2003). The purpose of this background review is not to synthesize the findings from all of the studies in a domain of inquiry, but rather to make a case for the specific study that it introduces: to identify the gaps, errors, or controversies that will be or were addressed in a study and to connect past research with the study proposed or just completed. Writers of such reviews are not obliged to detail the search strategies they used or the sampling frame for the studies they included.

Moreover, what makes this review "narrative" or "qualitative" is simply that words are used to conduct the review. This use of the terms *narrative* and *qualitative* should not be confused with the actual use of a form of narrative analysis or any one of a host of other specific qualitative methods (e.g., grounded theory) or techniques (e.g., qualitative thematic or content analysis) to study studies (Jones, 2004). Unfortunately, the terms *narrative* and *qualitative* are still misused to refer to reviews of the literature that are deemed unsystematic or otherwise lacking in the scientific rigor claimed for statistical reviews, or quantitative meta-analysis.

In Contrast to the Narrative Overview

Although they may be systematic and exhaustive in the search, retrieval, and analysis procedures used, narrative overviews of research are often wider in scope than background reviews and always less penetrating than qualitative research syntheses as they merely survey the topics and methods used in a field of study. Such "résumé review(s)" (Kirkevold, 1997, p. 980) offer "efficient overview(s)" (p. 981) of the research literature for researchers and practitioners.

In Contrast to Syntheses of Quantitative Research Findings

Both qualitative and quantitative methods can be used to integrate the findings in reports of qualitative or quantitative studies. The differences between qualitative and quantitative synthesis studies lie in the kinds of methods typically used (i.e., meta-analysis in quantitative research synthesis and metasummary, metasynthesis, or modified meta-ethnography in qualitative research synthesis) and in the mode of interpretation (i.e., statistical inference versus case-bound and narrative explanation).

In Contrast to Secondary Analysis

In contrast to the emphasis in qualitative research synthesis on qualitative findings is the emphasis in qualitative secondary analysis and pooled case comparisons on qualitative data (Thorne, 1994; West & Oldfather, 1995). In secondary analysis, an original data set is subjected to re-analysis—or two or more such data sets generated in different studies are combined to constitute a new data set—to answer one or more new research questions. The primary data in qualitative secondary analysis studies are the "raw" interview, observation and other data generated in the field; the primary data in qualitative research synthesis studies are the findings generated from these raw data across a set of primary studies.

In Contrast to Within-Study and Within-Program of Research Syntheses

Qualitative research syntheses are also different from the syntheses of data constituting the findings (e.g., the grounded theories, phenomenologies, ethnographies, and the like) in primary qualitative studies. These within-study syntheses (i.e., findings in individual primary qualitative studies) are the primary data in qualitative research synthesis studies.

In the borderlands between secondary analyses of qualitative data, within-study syntheses, and qualitative research syntheses are projects in which investigators use qualitative research synthesis methods to synthesize or reinterpret findings within and across their own programs of research (McCormick, Rodney, & Varcoe, 2003; Sandelowski, 1995a). Both "raw" data and findings generated from those data may constitute the primary data in these borderland projects.

In Contrast to Metastudy

Qualitative research synthesis studies are different from other qualitative studies of studies, such as metastudy, largely by virtue of their focus on actually integrating research findings and the empirical/analytical treatment of these findings. As Noblit & Hare (1988) originally conceived it, meta-ethnography is a form of metastudy that entails the interpretive comparison of study findings, not the integration of them. As Paterson, Thorne, Canam, and Jillings (2001) described it, metastudy is most akin to operations used in intellectual history, history and philosophy of science, information science, and other disciplines focused on the evolution and critique of ideas and knowledge development and representation. Metastudies can be targeted toward the study of findings (meta-data analysis), methods (metamethod), and theories (metatheory) in a designated body of research, but they do not necessarily entail any actual combination, assimilation, or integration of them in the empirical/analytical sense. Instead, they constitute a critical/discursive engagement with them.

Metastudy is arguably better conceived, not as a form of research synthesis, but rather as a method for "rigorously and systematically deconstructing existing bodies of qualitative research findings" (Thorne, Jensen, Kearney, Noblit, & Sandelowski, 2004, p. 1357). These deconstructions may then be used as a foundation or context for research synthesis, as Greenhalgh and colleagues (2005) demonstrated in their delineation of the "metanarratives," or research traditions characterizing diffusion-of-innovation studies.

Qualitative research synthesis studies have more limited empirical goals but greater immediate utility for practice than other studies of studies, such as metastudy. But metastudies aimed at the critical engagement between reviewers and, for example, the theories and methods characterizing a body of research offer an historical staging and explanatory context for qualitative research synthesis projects that assists reviewers to be more humble in their research integration claims. An example of a qualitative research synthesis study with a discursive disclaimer is our metasynthesis of motherhood in HIV-positive women in Sandelowski and Barroso (2003b). We discuss this role of metastudy in more detail in chapter 9.

Empirical versus Discursive Readings

As shown in Table 2.3, the empirical/analytical readings that characterize qualitative research synthesis write-ups can be distinguished from the critical/discursive readings that characterize qualitative metastudy works. In empirical/analytical readings, write-ups are viewed as indexes of studies and the outcomes of inquiry are viewed as findings that are, in turn, viewed as indexes of facts and feelings. Research syntheses are conceived here as empirically grounded and verifiable interpretations of the lived experiences of the research participants.

In contrast, in critical/discursive readings, write-ups of studies are conceived as historically and culturally contingent social products of unique encounters between researchers and research participants, and reviewers and texts, which reveal more about the experience of researching and the disciplinary commitments of writers than about the target experience itself. In contrast to the empirical/analytical view of research reports as indexes of studies, and of research outcomes as reasonably authentic accounts of facts and feelings, are views of them as narratives, cultural artifacts, social constructions, and discipline-specific discourses. (We discuss these distinctions further in chapter 5 as they relate to the conception of *data* and *findings* in qualitative research synthesis studies.)

Qualitative Research Synthesis as a Distinctive Enterprise

In summary, although it has features that overlap with other forms of inquiry, qualitative research synthesis—as depicted in this book—is characterized by the:

(a) systematic and comprehensive retrieval of all of the relevant reports of completed qualitative studies in a target domain of empirical inquiry;

(b) systematic use of qualitative and quantitative methods to analyze these reports;

(c) analytic and interpretive emphasis on the findings in these reports;

(d) systematic and appropriately eclectic use of qualitative methods to integrate the findings in these reports; and the

(e) use of reflexive accounting practices to optimize the validity of study procedures and outcomes.

Qualitative research synthesis is not easy to recognize as a distinctive enterprise because of the highly disparate entities that are presented as "critical," "integrative," "state of the art/science," or other reviews of the literature; qualitative research syntheses; qualitative or narrative methods to organize, analyze, or interpret bodies of literature; and as qualitative research itself (e.g., Dixon-Woods, Agarwal, Young, Jones, & Sutton, 2004; Weed, 2005; Whittemore, 2005). The distinctions we have drawn here are in the service of clarifying the focus of this book. They represent how we made sense of all the competing views of and claims concerning what are variously designated as critical, systematic, integrative, qualitative, narrative, and/or quantitative reviews of the literature or qualitative syntheses. We hope they help you make sense of them and to draw your own distinctions, as this will be necessary for you to determine the kind of project you want to conduct and to locate your unique project for your readers.

FORMULATING PURPOSE AND RATIONALE

Like primary qualitative studies, qualitative research synthesis studies usually begin with a research problem that can be addressed by research synthesis. Arguably the most common problem generating qualitative research synthesis projects is the proliferation of studies addressing a common experience, but lack of direction for interpreting or using their findings. Accordingly, a common purpose of a research synthesis study is to sum up the knowledge generated in an area in order to draw conclusions directly relevant to practice or chart directions for future research. Another example of a research problem is the proliferation of primary studies in a common area with apparently discrepant findings. The purpose of a research synthesis study might, therefore, be to account for or to resolve these discrepancies. Other purposes may include clarifying or modeling the relationships among research variables, defining the conditions under which a phenomenon appears, explaining or providing a context for the findings of primary quantitative research or research syntheses, or mapping knowledge fields.

As you formulate your objectives, you will also have to decide whether they are best met in one synthesis study, or a program of studies. For example, if your ultimate aim is to explain how gender shapes the experience of an illness, an explicit comparison is warranted of women and men. Describing only women's or only men's experiences will not satisfy the objective of explaining gender if women's experiences are not specifically juxtaposed with men's in the analysis and interpretation of research findings. Accordingly, you may determine that you have the human and material resources to integrate findings from qualitative studies of women with the target illness, of men with the target illness, and from studies that address the experiences of both women and men. Or you may decide on a program of research that includes first a synthesis of findings concerning women, second a synthesis of findings concerning men, and finally a synthesis of these syntheses aimed at comparing one group with the other.

A key issue in conceiving your project is to balance the specific research synthesis mandate to consider all of the research reports in a target area with the general qualitative research warrant to conduct in-depth analyses of every one of these reports. Qualitative research mandates that samples not be so large as to preclude intensive study. Indeed, whereas a threat to the validity of a qualitative research synthesis study is not to have conducted a sufficiently exhaustive search (see chapter 3), a threat to the validity of any qualitative study is to have a sample size so large that it exceeds the ability of researchers to conduct the intensive analysis of particulars that is the hallmark of excellent qualitative research. As you conceive your project, you must consider how to fulfill your research purpose with a study that is neither so limited nor so ambitious that its findings will be insignificant or superficial. No matter what research problem you choose, you must make a case that it exists, for whom it exists, and that it is significant enough to warrant the research synthesis study you want to conduct. Qualitative research synthesis studies are resource-intensive and, therefore, demand that you defend their expense by demonstrably linking the purpose of your study to a significant research problem.

ACCOMMODATING QUALITATIVE RESEARCH SYNTHESIS STUDIES TO AVAILABLE RESOURCES

Qualitative research synthesis studies require a diverse array of resources. As you formulate your project, you will need to determine what resources it will demand and what resources are available to you. This means you will have to estimate the amount and nature of the literature you will likely have to retrieve and analyze, determine the databases to which you have access, and assess the overall comprehensiveness of your library. If you do not have optimal access to the literature you will need to conduct a worthy qualitative research synthesis study, you will have to consider whether you can obtain access to the resources of another university or library or collaborate with a colleague who has access to such resources. Again, the most important threat to the validity of any research synthesis effort is to fail to conduct a sufficiently exhaustive search.

Research, Clinical, and Information Expertise

Qualitative research synthesis studies benefit from having a team of researchers and consultants with research, clinical, and information expertise. Having research, clinical, and information expertise will optimize the theoretical, pragmatic, and ethical validity of the research synthesis process and product; the evidence syntheses you produce will be credible as science and able to be translated into material form for practice (e.g., clinical guideline, appraisal tool). Research experts should possess the connoisseurship that comes with a wide-ranging knowledge of and skills in using qualitative methods. Qualitative research synthesis studies are for qualitative research connoisseurs and pluralists, not for methodological novices or purists with unwavering commitments to only one method or rigid ideas about how to implement methods (Johnson, Long, & White, 2001). Clinical experts should possess knowledge of the practice area that is the topical focus of the synthesis project and of ways to translate the synthesis itself into clinically useful knowledge. Information experts should have a wide-ranging knowledge of search strategies and sources, especially those related to qualitative research, and skill in the use of information technology. Harris (2005) described the critical role librarians play as expert searchers on research synthesis teams.

You will also want to consider employing research assistants with the intellectual, organizational, and technological skills, and the curiosity and perseverance to perform highly detail-oriented tasks under your direction, such as searching and retrieving relevant literature. They will have to be meticulous about documenting searches, including the databases and terms they used, and any revisions they made during the search. Once the relevant studies are retrieved, they can assist with managing the voluminous amount of text you will have, creating data displays, and analyzing findings.

Time and Labor

Qualitative research synthesis studies are time- and labor-intensive. They require you to set time aside from your other responsibilities for the intensive analysis each primary study demands. These projects are also time-sensitive. The time it takes to integrate a set of findings must not be so long as to preclude a timely integration. Because of the speed of advances in health care, findings may no longer be relevant, or worth integrating. Indeed, you will want to include the temporal relevance of studies as an inclusion criterion (see chapter 3).

Material Resources

The validity of any research synthesis project rests in part on having retrieved all relevant reports of studies in a target domain. Besides the costs of printing (online articles), copying (articles retrieved from the library), and inter-library loan fees to retrieve reports, you may have to purchase theses and dissertations. In the Metasynthesis Project, we had to purchase most of the theses and dissertations (in 2000–2002, at a cost of $31 per item) because we could not obtain them through interlibrary loan. The purchase of such reports is an important factor to consider in your budget as you work to accommodate study purposes to resources and consider seeking funds for your project.

Research synthesis studies also require sufficient supplies of paper and diskettes or CD-ROMs for scanning, computing, copying, printing, and backup storage. Other material resources to consider include computer hardware with sufficient space to accommodate the volume of data you will be scanning and the additional data you will be producing in the course of analyzing reports and integrating research findings. A good scanner with an excellent optical character recognition program and a photocopy machine are crucial items to have. You should also consider the software you will need to track the results of the search process, to manage your data, and to assist with analyzing them. For example, you should purchase a reference manager, such as EndNote® (http://www.endnote.com/) or ProCite® (http://www.procite.com/).

You may also want to consider purchasing a qualitative text management program, such as ATLAS.ti or NVivo. Although computer-assisted qualitative data analysis software (CAQDAS) allows efficient retrieval of information grouped together (or coded) and assists analysis, and may be especially useful in team research, word processing and other software enabling graphical displays may be all that is required. Researchers often have expectations of CAQDAS that it cannot meet and have been misled into thinking its relatively meager capabilities can serve as a frame for analysis (MacMillan & Koenig, 2004). Researchers can be taken in by the "veneer of objectivity they confer" (Sandelowski, 1995b, p. 205) and by the "wow factor" (MacMillan & Koenig, 2004) that seems to be generated by any technological innovation.

Accordingly, as you proceed with your synthesis study, be careful not to mistake a research tool for the research itself, or operating a program for analyzing a data set. Be careful not to permit your analytic decisions to be directed by and, therefore, restricted to what a program can do. They should be restricted only to what you can do.

TABLE 2.1 Comparison of Reviews of Literature, Secondary Analysis, and Studies of Studies

Type of review or study	Background review	Narrative overview	Qualitative secondary analysis/ pooled case comparison	Studies of studies		
				Research synthesis studies		Metastudies
Purpose	To stage proposed or completed study. To link proposed or completed study to other research in or out of the field. To make a case for the proposed or completed study	To inventory or survey topics addressed, & methods used, in a selected domain of inquiry	To reanalyze data collected in one or more primary studies	To produce a qualitative synthesis of research findings	To produce a quantitative synthesis of research findings	To interpret one or more elements of studies comprising a domain of inquiry
Primary data	Range of literature in one or more domains of inquiry, including qualitative & quantitative research reports, theoretical & clinical papers, memoirs &	Reports of empirical qualitative and/or quantitative research	Original qualitative data	Qualitative and/or quantitative research findings	Qualitative and/or quantitative research findings	Research traditions: Theories Methods Samples Findings

(continued)

TABLE 2.1 Comparison of Reviews of Literature, Secondary Analysis, and Studies of Studies (*Continued*)

Type of review or study	Background review	Narrative overview	Qualitative secondary analysis/pooled case comparison	Studies of studies	
				Research synthesis studies	Metastudies
Primary data (*con't*)	autobiographies & other reviews of literature				
Reading	Empirical/analytical	Empirical/analytical	Empirical/analytical, Critical/discursive	Empirical/analytical, Critical/discursive	Critical/discursive
Logic	Chain of reasoning	Catalog	Reframing	Aggregation, Integration	Critique, Interpretive comparison
Methods	Selected review of literature	Systematic review	Any qualitative or quantitative methods	Qualitative metasynthesis (or, meta-data analysis), Modified meta-ethnography, Systematic narrative review, Qualitative metasummary, Quantitative meta-analysis	Meta-theory, Meta-method, Meta-ethnography, Meta-narrative

Method references	Hart, 1998	Kirkevold, 1997	Heaton, 2004 Thorne, 1994	Britten et al., 2002 Sandelowski & Barroso, 2003c	Cooper, 1998 Sandelowski & Barroso, 2003a	Greenhalgh et al., 2005 Noblit & Hare, 1988 Paterson et al., 2001
Published examples	See review of literature in any report of empirical research	McKevitt et al., 2004	Reinharz, 1993	Campbell et al., 2003 Donald et al., 2005 Sandelowski & Barroso, 2003b	Hodges et al., 2005 Sandelowski et al., 2004	Paterson et al., 2003 Thorne, Joachim et al., 2002 Thorne, Paterson et al., 2002

TABLE 2.2 Comparison of Synthesis Outcomes in Qualitative Inquiry by Location

Location	Within primary study	Within single program of research	Across studies in a target domain
Synthesis outcomes	Grounded theories Ethnographies Phenomenologies . . . And the like	Reinterpretations Theories Conceptual maps . . . And the like	Qualitative metasummaries Qualitative metasyntheses Modified meta-ethnographies

TABLE 2.3 Empirical/Analytical Versus Critical/Discursive Readings of Qualitative Research Write-Ups

	Empirical/Analytical	Critical/Discursive
View of research write-up	Report, index of study	Writing practice, rhetoric, cultural artifact
View of inquiry outcomes	Research findings; indexes of facts and feelings	Narratives, discourses, moral accounts, social constructions
Orientation to language	Neutral vehicle of communication	Practice constituting communication
Orientations to data and findings	Data-based	Data as constructed
Logic of reading	Reading lines	Reading into and between the lines; over-reading; reading for silences, what is missing; rewriting
	Reducing text	Complicating text
View of researcher/ reviewer	Reporter/communicator	Representative of disciplinary, cultural group; narrator, information or impression manager
	Humanist stable self	Post-human virtual, plastic, polyvocal selves
View of research synthesis	Data-based and verifiable index of findings across a set of reports	Discourse Not possible to synthesize Not desirable to synthesize

REFERENCES

Britten, N., Campbell, R., Pope, C., Donovan, J., Morgan, M., & Pill, R. (2002). Using meta-ethnography to synthesize qualitative research: A worked example. *Journal of Health Services Research & Policy, 7,* 209–215.

Campbell, R., Pound, P., Pope, C., Britten, N., Pill, R., Morgan, M., et al. (2003). Evaluating meta-ethnography: A synthesis of qualitative research on lay experiences of diabetes and diabetes care. *Social Science & Medicine, 56,* 671–684.

Cooper, H. (1998). *Synthesizing research: A guide for literature reviews* (3rd ed.). Thousand Oaks, CA: Sage.

Dixon-Woods, M., Agarwal, S., Young, B., Jones, D., & Sutton, A. (2004). *Integrative approaches to qualitative and quantitative evidence.* London: National Health Service, Health Development Agency (Retrieved March 14, 2006, from http://www.med.umich.edu/csp/Course%20materials/ Summer%202005/Goold_Integrative_Approaches.pdf).

Donald, M., Dower, J., & Kavanagh, D. (2005). Integrated versus non-integrated management and care for clients with co-occurring mental health and substance use disorders: A qualitative systematic review of randomised controlled trials. *Social Science & Medicine, 60,* 1371–1383.

Doyle, L. H. (2003). Synthesis through meta-ethnography: Paradoxes, enhancements, and possibilities. *Qualitative Research, 3,* 321–345.

Greenhalgh, T., Robert, G., Macfarlane, F., Bate, P., Kyriakidou, O., & Peacock, R. (2005). Storylines of research in diffusion of innovation: A meta-narrative approach to systematic review. *Social Science & Medicine, 61,* 417–430.

Harris, M. R. (2005). The librarian's role in the systematic review process: A case study. *Journal of the Medical Library Association, 93,* 81–87.

Hart, C. (1998). *Doing a literature review: Releasing the social science research imagination.* London: Sage.

Heaton, J. (2004). *Reworking qualitative data.* London: Sage.

Hodges, L. J., Humphris. G. M., & Macfarlane, G. (2005). A meta-analytic investigation of the relationship between the psychological distress of cancer patients and their carers. *Social Science & Medicine, 60,* 1–12.

Johnson, M., Long, T., & White, A. (2001). Arguments for "British pluralism" in qualitative health research. *Journal of Advanced Nursing, 33,* 243–249.

Jones, K. (2004). Mission drift in qualitative research, or moving toward a systematic review of qualitative studies, moving back to a more systematic narrative review. *The Qualitative Report, 9*(1), 95–112. Retrieved August 29, 2004, from www.nova.edu/ssss/ QR/QR9-1/jones.pdf

Kirkevold, M. (1997). Integrative nursing research: An important strategy to further the development of nursing science and nursing practice. *Journal of Advanced Nursing, 25,* 977–984.

MacMillan, K., & Koenig, T. (2004). The wow factor: Preconceptions and expectations for data analysis software in qualitative research. *Social Science Computer Review, 22,* 179–186.

McCormick, J., Rodney, P., & Varcoe, C. (2003). Reinterpretations across studies: An approach to meta-analysis. *Qualitative Health Research, 13,* 933–944.

McKevitt, C., Redfern, J., Mold, F., & Wolfe, C. (2004). Qualitative studies of stroke: A systematic review. *Stroke, 35,* 1499–1505.
Noblit, G. W., & Hare, R. D. (1988). *Meta-ethnography: Synthesizing qualitative studies.* Newbury Park, CA: Sage.
Paterson, B., Canam, C., Joachim, G., & Thorne, S. (2003). Embedded assumptions in qualitative studies of fatigue. *Western Journal of Nursing Research, 25,* 119–133.
Paterson, B. L., Thorne, S. E., Canam, C., & Jillings, C. (2001). *Meta-study of qualitative health research: A practical guide to meta-analysis and meta-synthesis.* Thousand Oaks, CA: Sage.
Poirier, S., & Ayres, L. (1997). Endings, secrets, and silences: Overreading in narrative inquiry. *Research in Nursing & Health, 20,* 551–557.
Reinharz, S. (1993). Empty explanations for empty wombs: An illustration of secondary analysis of qualitative data. In M. Schratz (Ed.), *Qualitative voices in educational research* (pp. 157–178). London: Falmer Press.
Sandelowski, M. (1995a). A theory of the transition to parenthood of infertile couples. *Research in Nursing & Health, 18,* 123–132.
Sandelowski, M. (1995b). On the aesthetics of qualitative research. *Image: Journal of Nursing Scholarship, 27,* 205–209.
Sandelowski, M. (2001). Real qualitative researchers do not count: The use of numbers in qualitative research. *Research in Nursing & Health, 24,* 230–240.
Sandelowski, M., & Barroso, J. (2003a). Creating metasummaries of qualitative findings. *Nursing Research, 52,* 226–233.
Sandelowski, M., & Barroso, J. (2003b). Motherhood in the context of maternal HIV infection. *Research in Nursing & Health, 26,* 470–482.
Sandelowski, M., & Barroso, J. (2003c). Toward a metasynthesis of qualitative findings on motherhood in HIV-positive women. *Research in Nursing & Health, 26,* 153–170.
Sandelowski, M., Lambe, C., & Barroso, J. (2004). Stigma in HIV-positive women. *Journal of Nursing Scholarship, 36,* 123–129.
Thorne, S. (1994). Secondary analysis in qualitative research: Issues and implications. In J. M. Morse (Ed.), *Critical issues in qualitative research methods* (pp. 263–279). Thousand Oaks, CA: Sage.
Thorne, S., Jensen, L., Kearney, M. H., Noblit, G., & Sandelowski, M. (2004). Qualitative metasynthesis: Reflections on methodological orientation and ideological agenda. *Qualitative Health Research, 14,* 1342–1365.
Thorne, S., Joachim, G., Paterson, B., & Canam, C. (2002). Influence of the research frame on qualitatively derived health science. *International Journal of Qualitative Methods, 1*(1), Article 1. Retrieved March 14, 2003, from www.ualberta.ca/~ijqm/
Thorne, S., Paterson, B., Acorn, S., Canam, C., Joachim, G., & Jillings, C. (2002). Chronic illness experience: Insights from a metastudy. *Qualitative Health Research, 12,* 437–452.
Weed, M. (2005). "Meta-Interpretation": A method for the interpretive synthesis of qualitative research. *Forum: Qualitative Social Research, 6*(1), Article 37. Retrieved March 14, 2006, from http://www.qualitative-research.net/fqs-texte/1-05/05-1-37-e.htm

West, J., & Oldfather, P. (1995). Pooled case comparison: An innovation for cross-case study. *Qualitative Inquiry, 1,* 452–464.

Whittemore, R. (2005). Combining evidence in nursing research: Methods and implications. *Nursing Research, 54,* 56–62.

CHAPTER THREE

Searching For and Retrieving Qualitative Research Reports

Valid research syntheses depend on the comprehensive retrieval of all research reports relevant to a domain of study. The most important threat to the validity of any research synthesis—whether of qualitative or quantitative findings—is the failure to conduct a sufficiently exhaustive search. In this chapter, we focus on issues related to locating qualitative research reports. We assume you already have a general acquaintance and facility with searching and particularly with using electronic databases.

SETTING PARAMETERS FOR THE SEARCH

Recall and *precision* are the most commonly used performance measures in information retrieval. Recall is the percent of relevant documents in the database that have been retrieved. Precision is the percent of documents that have been retrieved that are relevant. Searches may, thus, be categorized as high-recall searches, in which most or all of the documents on a topic are retrieved, and high-precision searches, in which the set of documents retrieved consists of a smaller number of predominantly relevant documents (Losee, 2000; Marchionini, 1995). Ideally, research synthesis studies should emphasize recall over precision to ensure an exhaustive search.

After determining the initial purpose of your research synthesis study, you must set the initial topical (what), population (who), temporal (when), and methodological (how) parameters for your search. These parameters will constitute the inclusion criteria for your project and clarify what studies should be excluded. These settings are subject to change as you encounter research reports and become more familiar with the landscape of your chosen area of study.

Setting Topical Parameters

Here you choose what you will study. The what may specify a disease or diagnosis (e.g., HIV infection, positive prenatal diagnosis), a facet of experience (e.g., motherhood in the context of maternal HIV infection, decision making after positive prenatal diagnosis), an event (e.g., pregnancy termination), or any other clearly defined topic. Indeed, you cannot proceed with your search without having a working definition of your topic. For example, in the Metasynthesis Project, we initially defined motherhood as encompassing the decision to become a mother and the experiences of actually being a mother. We initially defined positive prenatal diagnosis as any diagnosis of a fetal impairment during pregnancy.

As you retrieve the reports that will become part of your study, you will refine your definitions. For example, we encountered a few findings about HIV-positive mothers of adult children and decided to amend our definition of motherhood as encompassing the decision to become a mother and the experiences of actually being a mother to *minor children*. We encountered a report of a study of couples obtaining a positive maternal serum alpha-fetoprotein (MSAFP) test whose babies were found to be normal after amniocentesis. We decided this report was relevant because these couples were, for a period of time during pregnancy, under the influence of a positive diagnosis. Accordingly, we amended our working definition of *positive prenatal diagnosis* to include couples obtaining any diagnosis, or under suspicion of the existence, of a fetal impairment during pregnancy.

Because of the open nature of qualitative studies, it is commonplace for findings to be produced about topics researchers had not anticipated. Accordingly, another decision you will have to make in setting the topical boundaries for your search is whether you will include reports of studies with general research purposes (e.g., living with a disease) that are likely to contain findings concerning the specific topic of interest to you (e.g., adherence to medications, self-care), or only reports that specifically address your topic. Given the evolving nature of qualitative studies, a highly restricted topical search is likely to exclude findings relevant to your study. For example, 33 of the 56 research reports of studies with findings pertaining to motherhood in HIV-positive women in the Metasynthesis Project had research purposes other than the exploration of motherhood. If we had restricted our search only to reports of studies that had as their research purposes the exploration of some aspect of motherhood, we would not have known about the findings pertaining to motherhood contained in reports of studies related to other topics in the lives of HIV-positive women. Your knowledge of the research conducted in your target area will help you decide how expansive or restrictive your topical search should be.

Setting Population Parameters

Here you choose the people you will study. For example, we chose to focus on HIV-positive women of any race/ethnicity or nationality, but living in the United States. After we encountered reports including adolescent girls, we amended our definition to include HIV-positive *adult* women (i.e., older than 18) in order to clarify the line between studies of HIV-positive women and studies of HIV-positive children. We further decided to include only those studies conducted *with* HIV-positive women themselves, not studies *of* or *about* these women conducted with other persons, such as children, partners, or health care providers.

You must also defend your population parameters. For example, an explanation for limiting a study to HIV-positive *women,* as opposed to men, is that because gender is a key variable differentiating illness experience and women's experiences have been under-represented in studies of HIV infection, a separate focus on women is warranted. An explanation for limiting a study to HIV-positive women *living in the United States,* as opposed to any other country, is that the diversity in cultural norms, values, and health care delivery, and in attitudes toward and treatment of HIV/AIDS, preclude drawing conclusions about the lives of HIV-positive women that would be applicable in all national contexts. As we noted in chapter 2, if the purpose of a synthesis project is to draw conclusions about gender and/or nationality and HIV infection (i.e., gender and/or nationality and HIV infection are the topics, not just HIV infection), as opposed to women's or U.S. women's experiences only, it would have to include explicit comparisons between women and men and/or between U.S. women and women in one or more other national contexts. This may require retrieving research reports addressing these population parameters for concurrent or future synthesis.

Setting Temporal Parameters

Here you define the time frame for your research synthesis project. To address the two domains of research in the Metasynthesis Project, we decided to include all reports of qualitative studies conducted with HIV-positive women, and of all qualitative studies conducted with women or couples obtaining positive prenatal diagnosis, from the time the first such studies appeared, to a current endpoint. Once you have retrieved reports in the selected time frame, you must advise readers of both the retrieval and publication time frames for your search. For example, the HIV reports we retrieved between June 1, 2000, and December 31, 2002, were published or completed between 1991 (when the first qualitative study of women with HIV infection known to us to meet our inclusion criteria was completed) and 2002. (The long search time frame—June 1, 2000, to December 31, 2002—was to meet the requirements of the Metasynthesis Project, a methods study.) The prenatal diagnosis reports we retrieved between December 1, 2002, and March 31, 2003, were published or completed between 1984 and 2002.

Time is a key parameter because of ongoing advancements in all practice fields (especially health care) and the need to have a timely (and not overly time-intensive) synthesis relevant to contemporary practice. For example, protease inhibitors and highly active antiretroviral therapy entered clinical practice in 1996, during the period of time covered by the HIV reports, or 1991–2002. This therapy contributed to the transformation of HIV infection from a fatal to a chronic disease; from a disease people die from to one they can live with. During the time period covered by the prenatal diagnosis reports, 1984–2002, technological innovations allowed earlier diagnosis, and access to abortion in the United States was further restricted. Time is also a key parameter in the appraisal of research reports as it must be accounted for in the synthesis of research findings (see chapter 4).

Setting Methodological Parameters

Because qualitative research synthesis studies are about integrating qualitative research findings, you must be able to differentiate qualitative research from other kinds of studies and from other things designated as *qualitative* (Grant, 2004). Defining qualitative research will not necessarily be easy because highly disparate entities are all referred to as qualitative research (Morales, 1995), and because researchers often do not explicitly name their methods in their reports. Indeed, the only indication of qualitative method might be a citation to a reference by a scholar associated with it, as when an author cites Van Manen's (1990) text on hermeneutic phenomenology as a resource, but never mentions this method anywhere in the report. Moreover, finding relevant qualitative studies is especially challenging because of the "multidisciplinary pedigree of the qualitative research literature" (Barbour & Barbour, 2003, p. 183). This pedigree requires searching databases and print collections representing literature across the sciences, humanities, and arts and the development of an extensive list of search terms to capture the diverse ways that qualitative research is labeled and indexed (or to overcome the fact that it is neither named nor indexed as qualitative research).

Several factors complicate the problem of defining and, therefore, locating relevant qualitative research reports. Probably the most important one is that "qualitative research" is conducted by scholars with highly diverse disciplinary affiliations. A second complicating factor is the tendency to conflate qualitative research with qualitative data. No matter what the discipline, qualitative research is generally presented in didactic texts as a distinctive and all-encompassing gestalt for inquiry. Great care is typically given to defining the ontological, epistemological, and methodological standpoints of practitioners of qualitative research, with a view to demonstrating their difference from quantitative research. In contrast, the term *qualitative data* is used to refer to anything involving words, which, in effect, excludes nothing in the landscape of human inquiry. Indeed, any paper-and-pencil data collection instrument is arguably qualitative as it involves words and/or pictures, and it is words that investigators use to interpret the results of statistical tests and to persuade readers of their quantitative significance (Gephart, 1988).

A third complicating factor related to the conflation of qualitative research with qualitative data is the increasing tendency to view qualitative and quantitative research as mixable and even as interchangeable (Swanborn, 1996; Valsiner, 2000). This move toward peaceful co-existence and the eliding of difference has resulted in a dizzying array of highly divergent and often overlapping conceptualizations of qualitative research and so-called mixed methods research involving qualitative methods. Indeed, in recent years, there has been an increasing number of investigator claims to having conducted mixed methods studies in which qualitative data or qualitative data collection and/or analysis techniques were used, but in which there is no evidence in the research report of the use of any qualitative method. This claim seems to have become a rhetorical appeal not only to methodological fashion, but also to methodological ecumenicism, expertise, and rigor (Sandelowski, 2003b).

The reports most troubling to the definition of qualitative research are of studies that meet neither the probability sampling and psychometric requirements of quantitative research, nor the purposeful sampling and interpretive requirements of qualitative research. (We further describe these types of reports in chapter 5.) As they comprise a significant proportion of contemporary research in the practice disciplines, these reports will compel you to differentiate between reports of qualitative research and: (a) reports of research that merely contain verbal data, or more verbal than numerical data; (b) reports of research in which techniques for data collection (e.g., open-ended interviews) or analysis (e.g., content analysis) commonly viewed as qualitative were used to produce only surface treatments of data; and (c) reports of quantitative descriptive research, including surveys.

While setting the methodological parameters for a qualitative research integration study, you should try to ensure that the label *qualitative research* not be "co-opted" for studies that, albeit informative, offer no more than another "surface understanding" of human experience (Metz, 2000, p. 67) or that demand no more of researchers than the ability to listen and record. The label *qualitative research* should be reserved for those studies that demonstrate researchers' recognition of the ephemeral, complicated, and situated nature of events, including the research act itself. Here is our working definition of qualitative research.

> *Qualitative research* is an umbrella term for an array of attitudes toward and strategies for conducting inquiry that are aimed at discerning how human beings understand, experience, interpret, and produce the social world (Mason, 1996). Qualitative research encompasses richly detailed descriptions and in-depth, particularized interpretations of persons and the social, linguistic, material, and other practices and events that shape their lives and are shaped by them. Qualitative research typically includes, but is not limited to, discerning the perspectives of these persons, or what is often referred to as the actor's or emic point of view. Although both philosophically and methodologically a highly diverse entity, qualitative research is marked by certain defining imperatives that include a case-orientation (as opposed to variable-orientation) to analysis, sensitivity to cultural and historical context, and reflexive accounting practices to optimize validity. In its many guises in health research, qualitative research is a form of empirical inquiry that typically entails: (a) some form of purposeful sampling for information-rich cases; (b) in-depth and open-ended interviews, lengthy participant/field observations, and/or document or artifact study; and (c) techniques for analysis and interpretation of data that move beyond the data generated and their surface appearances (Sandelowski, 2003a, pp. 893–894).

To complete our setting of methodological parameters in the Metasynthesis Project, we specifically excluded: (a) qualitative studies in which no human subjects participated (e.g., discourse or content analyses of media representations of HIV-positive women); (b) mixed methods studies in which qualitative findings could not be separated from quantitative findings; (c) mixed sample qualitative studies in which findings about the target population could not be separated from those about other populations (e.g., HIV-negative women, women with cancer, couples obtaining negative diagnoses); (d) alternative-style qualitative research presentations containing no extractable findings (e.g., poems, plays, auto-ethnographies); and (e) journalistic or other nonresearch, albeit narrative, accounts.

BROWSING AND BERRY-PICKING

Once you have set the initial parameters for your synthesis project, you must decide where you will search for reports of studies within those parameters. With the proliferation of information sources and information technology, you will have to choose from among many types of sources and search techniques. Advances in information technology should not deter you from pursuing traditional information sources, such as personal contacts and research conferences. Other important information sources are the web sites of professional organizations, government institutions, and collections of systematic reviews, such as the Association of Nurses in AIDS Care (ANAC), the Association of Women's Health, Obstetric, and Neonatal Nurses (AWHONN), the National Institutes of Health, and the Cochrane Library.

Bates (1989) used the metaphors of browsing and berry-picking to describe search strategies. Browsing the literature is a strategy useful to stimulate thinking and to help searchers get the lay of the land. Browsing is also an important component of berry-picking. Berry-picking is a dynamic and iterative process (akin to qualitative inquiry itself) whereby searchers continually modify the search terms for a query, as well as the query itself. Queries are satisfied, not by a single final retrieved set of reports, but rather by a series of selections searchers make of individual references and bits of information at each stage of the search. A bit-at-a-time retrieval of this sort is called berry-picking. Just as a berry-picker meanders (as opposed to moving in a straight line) through the bushes looking for clumps of berries, the searcher wanders through the information forest, changing direction as needed to follow up on various leads and shifts in thinking. The key is to keep track of and account for these shifts.

Bates (1989) described six berry-picking strategies. All six strategies should be used systematically, with all leads to relevant literature pursued as they are generated from each one.

Footnote Chasing

Also called backward chaining and the ancestry approach (Cooper, 1998, p. 56), this technique involves following up on references listed in literature on the selected topic of study. In the Metasynthesis Project, we reviewed thousands of citations from the reference lists of relevant research reports, and other articles, books, anthologies, and conference and technical reports. One way to know you have conducted a comprehensive search is when you achieve citation redundancy; you reach a point where you have perused every potentially relevant reference and no new relevant references appear.

Citation Searching

Also called forward chaining and the descendency approach (Cooper, 1998, p. 62), citation searching begins with a citation. Searchers use a citation database, such as the *Social Sciences Citation Index,* to find out what other works contain the citation and thereby leap forward in their search. Searchers can use the titles of reports known to be relevant to locate other potentially relevant reports, which, in some databases, are indexed as "related works."

Table 3.1 shows what reports were cited in each of the HIV reports included in the Metasynthesis Project. Because it usually takes time for a work to disseminate widely, the fruitfulness of this approach is dependent on whether a work is available (and to what degree) to be cited in more recent works. A significant proportion of the reports listed in Table 3.1 are not published works and were, therefore, more difficult to access. Access to these sources was further impeded because authors of reports derived from their theses or dissertations did not cite these works.

Even when available, reports may remain uncited (Campbell et al., 2003). As shown in Table 3.1, authors often did not cite each other even when reports could have been located. Factors that may account for this include inadequate search resources and strategies and the still-prevalent but erroneous idea that qualitative research ought to be conducted naively and the literature review in the target area delayed. This unfortunate state of affairs undermines the utility of qualitative research; studies that address research questions that have already been answered, or that offer formulations of events as innovative when they are not, are endlessly repeated (and not even explicitly for replication purposes).

Journal Runs and Hand Searching

Here searchers identify journals central to the field of study and search each one systematically by hand. Such a technique guarantees complete recall within the journals selected. To locate HIV reports, we hand-searched *Qualitative Health Research,* the premier journal in qualitative health research, and the *Journal of the Association of Nurses in AIDS Care,* the flagship journal of the Association of Nurses in AIDS Care. To locate prenatal diagnosis reports, we hand-searched *Qualitative Health*

Research, Fetal Diagnosis, a journal devoted solely to the selected topic; *Birth,* a journal devoted to research in all facets of childbearing; and *JOGNN: Journal of Obstetric, Gynecologic, & Neonatal Nursing,* the flagship journal of the Association of Women's Health, Obstetric, and Neonatal Nurses.

Hand searches are also critical to finding relevant studies in anthologies. Book chapters are typically not indexed or described in sufficient detail in electronic databases. Such searches can also serve to evaluate the accuracy of electronic searching. For example, to locate prenatal diagnosis reports, we searched our own collection of books in this area and located chapters containing reports relevant to the topic. When several of these books failed to surface in the initial searches of electronic databases, we knew we had not yet found the right search terms. We revised our terms until these previously excluded reports appeared. The mistake we made was to add the word *women* to the search. As prenatal diagnosis unavoidably involves women, using *women* as a search term here was not only unnecessary but also served to exclude relevant literature. This event also underscored for us the importance of having research synthesis studies conducted by reviewers who know the topical domain selected and are likely to own key works in the field.

Area Scanning

This strategy refers to browsing materials that are physically colocated with materials retrieved earlier in a search. For example, once we had identified books on HIV-positive women and prenatal diagnosis, we scanned the shelf locations of these books to find other books that might be of interest to us. We also used this strategy to locate materials electronically co-located, by searching the electronic card catalog of our library system for materials included under subject headers such as "women and HIV," "prenatal diagnosis," "fetal diagnosis," "reproductive technology," and "motherhood." We knew from our knowledge of the literature on HIV-positive women and on prenatal diagnosis that anthologies on motherhood could have relevant reports.

Another means to find materials electronically colocated is to follow the link to "related works" offered in some electronic databases.

Author Searching

Based on relevant publications found previously, this strategy entails searching every database by the names of authors of relevant reports to ascertain whether they completed other works on the same topic. We found this technique especially useful for locating the theses and dissertations from which many of the published reports were derived. As we noted previously, the authors of published works tended not to cite these works.

Subject Searches in Electronic Bibliographic Databases

This technique is the most commonly used and involves searching electronic bibliographic databases likely to have relevant works in an area. We chose electronic bibliographic databases that were accessible to us, covered a wide range of disciplines, and that we knew or surmised would yield reports of relevant qualitative studies. Harris (2005) recommended searching MEDLINE first, because it is the largest and oldest database. Table 3.2 shows the list of databases—available through the library computer network at the University of North Carolina at Chapel Hill—we used between 2000–2003 to conduct the HIV and prenatal diagnosis searches. The search systems we used were primarily Ovid (Ovid Technologies, Inc.), SilverPlatter (SilverPlatter Information), and OCLC FirstSearch (OCLC Online Computer Library Center, Inc.). (SilverPlatter merged with Ovid in 2001.) We also worked closely with reference librarians and colleagues in the School of Information and Library Science with specialties in the health sciences. Enlisting the assistance of information specialists in the health sciences is vital to the most advantageous use of electronic databases (Harris, 2005).

The major difficulty in searching multiple databases, a must for retrieving all relevant qualitative studies, is that the searcher must know the different access and searching procedures required by each database. These procedures vary depending on the search system used. An example of this is the truncation symbol, which is an asterisk (*) in the U.S. National Library of Medicine's PubMed database, and a dollar sign ($) in the Ovid system. Truncation refers to the use of a special symbol that serves as a substitute for other characters. Attaching a truncation symbol to a word root pulls up variant forms of the word. There are even differences in capitalization and punctuation required to perform command syntax searching. Each database has its own unique subject term index (thesaurus), its own rules for searching (syntax), and its own style for data presentation (Harris, 2005).

Search Terms for Electronic Databases

The development of search terms appropriate to the area of interest and the database is essential for the effective use of electronic bibliographic databases. Some databases incorporate lists of official subject headings or controlled vocabulary terms that are available for searching. An example is the Medical Subject Headings, known as MeSH, used by the National Library of Medicine as indexing terms for MEDLINE and PubMed. Other databases work by natural language processing, which allows common or noncontrolled terms to be searched. Still other databases are searchable using both methods. In a controlled vocabulary database, the standardized search terms are on a list or thesaurus within the database. This list is not always readily apparent. In contrast, natural language processing allows the searcher to type in virtually any term or phrase and the database will attempt application.

Most databases will allow you to select the location or "field" to which the search terms should be applied (e.g., title, author, abstract, keywords, or *words anywhere*, meaning every textual piece related to a citation that is in the database). We used the *words anywhere* option in order to ensure a comprehensive search, which is a common technique in information retrieval (Coletti & Bleich, 2001; Marchionini, 1995; Meadow, Boyce & Kraft, 2000). However, using and exploding subject headings (in databases that allow this) often pulls up materials that would be missed by a *words anywhere* search. Accordingly, it may be necessary to use both techniques: a *words anywhere* search, and using and exploding subject headings.

Searchers have to become knowledgeable about the underlying mapping patterns of a database in order to manipulate search terms appropriately. Mapping is a relatively recent addition to the usual line of searching features. In mapping, the system offers additional terminology from the controlled vocabulary of a database in response to a search term entered by the user (Jasco, 1996). For example, in some databases, the search term *women* maps to *human female*. Human female includes *mothers, sisters, widows, daughters,* and *wives,* as well as *battered females, working women,* and *female criminals.* The database may be searching for keywords as provided by the author, the indexer, or contained in the title, abstract, or in the full text of the article. In Ovid-based MEDLINE and CINAHL, the subject headings presented during the mapping process can be selected or deselected, depending on the focus of the search and retrieval activity. Searchers must, therefore, manipulate their search terms according to the parameters of the systems used.

An especially challenging problem is retrieving research by the method used (Littleton, Marsalis, & Bliss, 2004) and, specifically, locating exclusively qualitative research reports. Part of the problem stems from the descriptive nature of the titles used for many qualitative studies, the variable information provided in abstracts, and the differences in indexing of these studies across databases (Evans, 2002). Some bibliographic databases do not index articles according to research methodology. As a search term, *qualitative research* yielded few relevant citations and many irrelevant ones, such as "qualitative" laboratory assays. The challenge was to find and combine search terms that spoke the language of each of the bibliographic databases while still representing qualitative research. When we first started searching, *qualitative research* in MEDLINE on Ovid mapped to a large number of subject headings, including *research, research design, nursing methodology research, nursing research, data interpretation, health services research, nursing,* and *myocardial infarction.* In 2003, MEDLINE added "qualitative research" as a Medical Subject Heading (MeSH) term. In Ovid-based CINAHL, *qualitative research* maps to the subject heading *qualitative studies,* and under this broad term are several narrower headings that describe specific types of qualitative research, such as *ethnographic research* and *phenomenological research.* To improve our chances of finding relevant research methods, we developed the list of search concepts, shown in Table 3.3. We included in this list terms such as "exploratory" and "content analysis," which do not signal exclusively qualitative research, but which are often the only terms used to refer to studies that may be qualitative. Where appropriate, we truncated terms to broaden the search.

An advancement that appeared after we completed our searches was the development of methodological search filters that sift out those studies using the research methods of interest. This greatly increases the precision of the search for qualitative studies without sacrificing the need for broad recall. Librarians developed these filters, shown in Table 3.4, for users of CINAHL, but they are not part of the CINAHL database or the Ovid interface. Although we used most of these same terms in our searches, CINAHL included the names of authors most often associated with certain qualitative methodologies. This will ensure a better search because, as we noted previously, sometimes the only reference to qualitative research contained in a report is a citation to the work of an author.

You may want to try using search terms to capture the thematic content likely to be the focus of qualitative research. For example, many health research domains, including HIV infection and prenatal diagnosis, are characterized by large numbers of studies in the biological, physiological, diagnostic, and other realms not typically addressed in qualitative studies. To avoid these, you may want to experiment with the addition of search terms such as *decision-making, psychological aspects,* and *sociocultural aspects.* Whether you maintain this search strategy will depend on the outcome of your trial.

Having a broad knowledge of related thematic lines is especially relevant to searching for qualitative studies in which the topical focus is a theme or concept, as opposed to specific persons or diseases or events. For example, you may be interested in integrating findings on "resilience." But limiting your search to this word alone will not result in a comprehensive search. Other related ideas, such as "inner strength," "hardiness," and "survivor(ship)," will have to be included in your search strategy. The results of your search using these terms will assist you to refine your search strategy to include, or deliberately exclude, other thematic lines you had not previously considered and, thereby, to reconsider the purpose of your study.

Time is also a factor in setting your search terms. Database producers make changes and additions to their controlled vocabularies, often on an annual basis. One example is the change over time in the names of diseases; what we now know as HIV infection was once known as GRID (gay-related immune deficiency), and the stage of illness prior to AIDS was known as ARC (AIDS-related complex). Another example is the move over time from the use of the term *compliance* to *adherence* to *concordance* to designate how and whether individuals take their medicines and do the treatments prescribed for them (Pound et al., 2005). Although these terms connote different ideas about agency and responsibility, they are often used loosely and interchangeably and must, therefore, be used as search terms in any synthesis project addressing whether, how, and under what circumstances people take their prescribed treatments.

An important principle in searching is that the limitations you place on your study should not necessarily be the limitations you place on your search strategy. In the Metasynthesis Project, we limited both our HIV and prenatal diagnosis studies to women or couples living in the United States, but no reliable means exists to retrieve reports of studies conducted only in the United States. Limiting searches to English-language literature will exclude studies conducted in the United States but reported in non-English language venues and will include studies conducted in other English-speaking countries. Similarly, nationality is a feature of journals, publishers, researchers, and participants, not just sites of data collection. Even if a database allows this limitation, using it will likely result in the exclusion of relevant reports.

The Dynamics of Electronic Bibliographic Databases

Electronic bibliographic databases are not stable entities yielding fixed search results. Each database offers numerous options for searching, and search features may change over time. Moreover, a database may exist one day as an independent entity and the next day be inaccessible, extinct, or incorporated into another database. Each database access provider has an information page with its parameters for updates and inclusion dates.

For example, in our library system, access to CD-ROM–based PsycLit was removed soon after we began our searches, leaving us access to an online database, PsycINFO. Early in our searching, journal citations that could be found in AIDSLINE, once an independent database, were incorporated into PubMed, the National Library of Medicine's database that includes MEDLINE. This change meant that our searches resulted in different outcomes. In addition, databases are updated at different intervals; they may be updated daily, quarterly, or only yearly, thereby contributing to a citation list that may not be current. You—the searcher—are also not a stable, unchanging entity. Variations in your activity, concentration, and fatigue levels will influence the amount of time spent conducting a search and, therefore, the quality of the search results. The main caveat here is that any search is a function of the capacities of the person who conducted it and the resources used by and available to that person during the specific hours they conducted the search.

One example of the complexity of searching options is that some databases, such as MEDLINE, CINAHL, and PsycINFO, have thesauri or controlled vocabularies that are divided hierarchically into broad and narrow terms. The narrower terms can be used to search for more specific information. Some databases also employ topical subheadings, which assist searchers to target particular aspects of a topic. These headings are the keys that unlock the medical literature (Coletti & Bleich, 2001). Decisions thus have to be made regarding which terms to use and how best to use them. For instance, in databases that have a hierarchical subject heading structure, the Ovid system allows searchers to "explode" a broad subject heading, thereby including all the narrower headings under it. Searchers may explore the list of subject headings to broaden the search and find related subjects, or "focus" a search term (to narrow the search) to look for citations in which the search term is a major point of the article. We chose to apply the "explode" feature, thus maximizing the use of MeSH headings. Searchers can use Boolean or other operators. Boolean operators allow the searcher to use set theory, which is commonly recognized in the form of a Venn diagram of overlapping circles indicating the "and," "or," and "not" functions that define the items that will be retrieved by a search. The use of special operators (e.g., proximity operators) is available in many databases, but some of the databases allow more flexible use than others. Expert-level searching generally entails searches that are conducted by professional search intermediaries who employ appropriate syntax, use of Boolean and other operators, and inclusion of desired delimiters or expanders for the search.

Although commonalities exist among databases, the vocabulary that is successful in searching for studies in one database will not necessarily be successful in another database. The search platform on which a database resides also influences searching and subsequent results. The same database provided by two different vendors can return different results from the same search, because searching features vary among database vendors. Minor idiosyncrasies, such as whether a comma should be used between an author's last name and first name (or initial), vary substantially among databases and can be frustrating to the searcher, in addition to providing an invalid search result. Few database systems return a message telling searchers that they have made a mistake in entering search terms. A "no records found" message may not reflect the absence of records so much as a system's inability to map the search terms used. If the search term is mapped to the "best judgment" of the programming within the database, totally irrelevant records may appear. The searcher may thus be faced with no citations or many irrelevant ones.

Although all the databases we used had characteristics that were supportive of our searches, we found Ovid to be the most useful search system for several reasons. Options in Ovid easily enable the searcher to see the hierarchy of subject headings, sometimes referred to as the "tree" structure, and relationships of individual search terms and to select or deselect the terms. Search terms can be expanded or focused in a variety of ways. Once visualized, we had some control in the selection/exclusion of a particular mapping. Merging of several individual search results in Ovid in order to form a comprehensive search for a concept helped to reduce the number of irrelevant citations. The subject headings that represent the indexing of each citation can be displayed, and these provide the searcher with a rich source of additional terms to use. We found this particularly helpful when developing an appropriate search term list. Ovid provides a clear error message when a searcher has made a mistake in handling search terms or applications. Ovid also permits the complex use of nested Boolean operators, and allows the user to save and email the results in a form that is friendly to importing directly into a reference manager database such as ProCite® or EndNote®.

FUGITIVE LITERATURE

Fugitive literature refers to potentially relevant works that are likely to escape the notice of searchers primarily because they are either not published or are published in venues not accessible via electronic databases. Among the most important of these works in qualitative research are Master's theses and doctoral dissertations, which their authors tend not to cite in subsequent reports of these studies. That is why searching by the names of authors whose reports are already included in your sample is a necessity. In addition, because they are produced with fewer space constraints than journal articles, theses and dissertations often contain more detail concerning methods and findings than the published reports derived from them. We located most of the theses and dissertations we were interested in through Dissertation Abstracts International (DAI) and, later, Digital Dissertations, although some of them appeared in other databases as well, such as PsycINFO or Sociological Abstracts.

DETERMINING RELEVANCE

Even after you have refined your search terms and techniques, you will likely still retrieve many citations that you will be unable to include or exclude on the basis of title and abstract alone. We found this to be especially true in the case of theses and dissertations. Because these works were often not available through interlibrary loan, we had to acquire them just to ascertain relevance. Jones (2004, p. 274) referred to this process as "sifting."

For the sake of efficiency and to avoid repeatedly evaluating the same citations appearing in different databases, you will have to develop a system to track the decisions you make about these citations. The process we used is shown in Figure 3.1. To optimize the validity of your search, at least two members of your research team should review all questionable citations and reach consensus on their disposition. Once a citation was obtained, we were sometimes able to exclude it based on the title alone. If we were unsure, we checked the abstract. A citation could then be excluded at this point as not meeting the criteria, or it could merit further investigation. If further investigation was warranted, the full report was obtained. At that point, the citation was included, excluded, or its status remained uncertain. Uncertain citations led to a negotiation of consensus on its status and further refinement and delineation of inclusion criteria. Once any report was finally included, we carefully examined it for the information properties that might lead us to locate other relevant reports. For example, we considered where we found the report and the key words used to describe it, and followed its related links.

MANAGING INFORMATION

Research synthesis projects typically generate volumes of information that require efficient management and cataloging. The foundation for ensuring valid procedures and results is the establishment of a clear audit trail documenting all procedural moves and decisions. The most important factor optimizing the validity of research synthesis studies is not the standardization of judgments, but rather the explication of the many judgments required to conduct these studies and produce research integrations (Nurius & Yeaton, 1987).

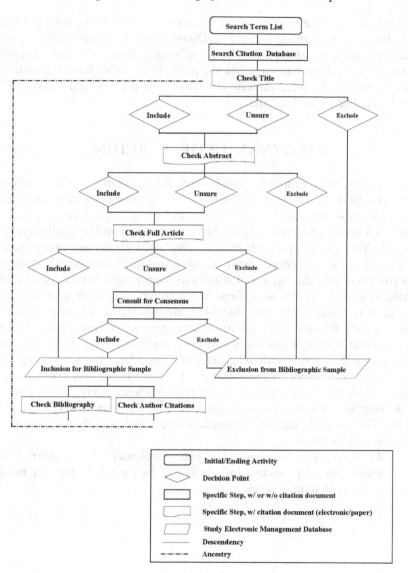

FIGURE 3.1 Search, retrieval, and validation process. Graphic symbols are drawn from Harris (1999, p. 156).

All the database systems we used supported the transfer of our search results to a printer and/or saving them on a disk or hard drive and, with a few exceptions, the transfer of results through e-mail. Ovid search results are also readily transferable into ProCite®, EndNote®, or other reference manager software packages, making management of the search results highly efficient and effective. We created several Access® databases for managing those citations that required more extensive tracking and handling, such as those located in Dissertation Abstracts. Information can be readily transferred between EndNote®, ProCite®, and Access® through several mechanisms. Via the publicly available PubMed system, our search results were directly downloadable through our university's ProCite® license at that time.

THE DYNAMICS OF SEARCHING

In summary, to accomplish a valid search for qualitative studies requires that you have the flexibility to match the constant change characterizing the contemporary search environment and technological innovation, as well as a broad understanding of the target domain and of qualitative research. You will find yourself revising your research purpose, your inclusion and exclusion criteria, your search terms, and your search strategy as you encounter the reports of studies in the area you have selected and, later, as you analyze these reports. You will have to decide at what temporal and substantive points you will be satisfied that you have completed your search. Because time lags always exist between the end of a search for a research integration study and the completion of the integration itself, you will have to decide whether you will update your search prior to submitting your report for publication. Even in the best of circumstances (e.g., where the publication of a research synthesis study occurs only a year after submission), the synthesis itself will be at least two years out of date. The need for comprehensiveness and timeliness should shape all your search decisions.

We invite you now to visit the supplement to chapter 3 at http://www.unc.edu/~msandelo/handbook/site/chapter3.html for modules on the searching process.

TABLE 3.1 Mutual Citations in Reports of Studies With HIV-Positive Women

Reports	Who cited the author?	Number of Reports Cited	Whom did the authors cite?	Number of Reports Cited
1991 Hutchison & Kurth	Armstrong, 1996 Bennett, 1997 Hassin, 1994 Hendrixson, 1996 Ingram, 1996 Ingram & Hutchinson, 1999a, 2000 Leenerts, 1997 Locher, 1995 Napravnik et al., 2000 Palyo, 1995 Rose, 1993 Sepples, 1996 Walsh, 2000	14	0	0
1992 Faithfull	0	0	0	0
1993 Andrews et al.	Armstrong, 1996 Bennett, 1997 Bunting & Seaton, 1999 Ciambrone, 2002 Dominguez, 1996 Faithfull, 1997 Gray, 1999 Ingram, 1996	20	0	0

(continued)

TABLE 3.1 Mutual Citations in Reports of Studies With HIV-Positive Women (*Continued*)

Reports	Who cited the author?	Number of Reports Cited	Whom did the authors cite?	Number of Reports Cited
1993 Andrews et al. *(cont'd)*	Ingram & Hutchinson, 1999a, 2000			
	Leenerts, 1997			
	Leenerts & Magilvy, 2000			
	Locher, 1995			
	Loriz-Lim, 1995			
	Palyo, 1995			
	Ross, 1994			
	Russell & Smith, 1999			
	Sepples, 1996			
	Walker, 1996			
	Walsh, 2000			
1993 Frey	Bell, 1997	2	0	0
	Walker, 1996			
1993 Rose	Bennett, 1997	11	Hutchison & Kurth, 1991	1
	Dominguez, 1996			
	Gramling et al., 1995			
	Ingram, 1996			
	Ingram & Hutchinson, 1999a, 2000			
	Leenerts, 1997			
	Leenerts & Magilvy, 2000			
	Ross, 1994			
	Russell & Smith, 1999			
	Woodard, 2002			

Study	Citing works			
1993 Salmon	Bell, 1997 Walsh, 2000	2	0	0
1993 Semple et al.	Bennett, 1997 Ciambrone, 1999 Dunbar et al., 1998 Goggin et al., 2001 Loriz-Lim, 1995 Russell & Smith, 1999 Schrimshaw et al., 2002 Van Servellen et al., 1998 Walsh, 2000 Winstead et al., 2002	11	0	0
1993 Tuchel & Feldman	0	0	0	0
1993 Weitz	Bennett, 1997 Ciambrone, 1999, 2001 Dozier, 1997 Marcenko & Samost, 1999	5	0	0
1994 Arnold	Walsh, 2000	1	0	0
1994 Bonifas	0	0	0	0
1994 Hassin	Bennett, 1997 Cameron, 2001 Stanley, 1999 Stevens & Doerr, 1997	4	Hutchison & Kurth, 1991	1

(continued)

TABLE 3.1 Mutual Citations in Reports of Studies With HIV-Positive Women (*Continued*)

Reports	Who cited the author?	Number of Reports Cited	Whom did the authors cite?	Number of Reports Cited
1994 Ross	0	0	Andrews et al., 1993 Rose, 1993	2
1995 Coward	Bennett, 1997 DeMarco et al., 1998 Haile et al., 2002 Leenerts, 1997 Leenerts & Magilvy, 2000 Moser et al., 2001 Sepples, 1996 Woodard & Sowell, 2001	8	0	0
1995 Gosling	0	0	0	0
1995 Kimberly et al.	Black & Miles, 2002 Schrimshaw et al., 2002 Serovich et al., 1998 Winstead et al., 2002	4	0	0
1995 Litwak et al.	Ciambrone, 1999	1	0	0
1995 Locher	0	0	Andrews et al., 1993 Hutchison & Kurth, 1991	2
1995 Loriz-Lim	0	0	Andrews et al., 1993 Semple et al., 1993	2

1995 Palyo	0	0	Andrews et al., 1993 Hutchison & Kurth, 1991	0	2
1995 Regan-Kubinski & Sharts-Hopko	Dunbar et al., 1998 Russell & Smith, 1999 Sepples, 1996 Van Loon, 2000	4	0	0	0
1995 Seals et al.	Ciambrone, 1999 Dunbar et al., 1998 Leenerts, 1998 Leenerts & Magilvy, 2000 Misener & Sowell, 1998 Russell & Smith, 1999 Valdez, 1999	7	0	0	0
1995 Tanner	0	0	0	0	0
1995 Wright	0	0	0	0	0
1996 Armstrong	0	0	Andrews et al., 1993 Hutchison & Kurth, 1991 Moneyham et al., 1996a, b	0	4
1996 Dominguez	0	0	Andrews et al., 1993 Rose, 1993	0	2
1996 Gramling et al.	0	0	Rose, 1993	0	1
1996 Hendrixson	0	0	Hutchison & Kurth, 1991	0	1

(continued)

TABLE 3.1 Mutual Citations in Reports of Studies With HIV-Positive Women (*Continued*)

Reports	Who cited the author?	Number of Reports Cited	Whom did the authors cite?	Number of Reports Cited
1996 Ingram	0	0	Andrews et al., 1993 Hutchison & Kurth, 1991 Rose, 1993	3
1996 Kass & Faden	0	0	0	0
1996a Moneyham et al.	Armstrong, 1996 Bennett, 1997 Black & Miles, 2002 Bunting & Seaton, 1999 Ciambrone, 1999 Ingram & Hutchinson, 1999a, b Leenerts, 1998 Leenerts et al., 1999 Leenerts & Magilvy, 2000 Schrimshaw et al., 2002 Valdez, 1999 Van Loon, 1996, 2000 Walsh, 2000 Woodard, 2002	16	0	0
1996b Moneyham et al.	Armstrong, 1996 Leenerts, 1998 Leenerts & Magilvy, 2000 Moser et al., 2001 Stanley, 1999	7	0	0

Study	Citations			Citations	
1996 Ritchie	Walsh, 2000; Woodard, 2002	0	0		0
1996 Sepples		0	0	Andrews et al., 1993; Coward, 1995; Hutchison & Kurth, 1991; Regan-Kubinski & Sharts-Hopko, 1995	4
1996 Sowell et al.	Bunting & Seaton, 1999; Leenerts, 1998; Leenerts et al., 1999; Leenerts & Magilvy, 2000; Misener & Sowell, 1998; Moser et al., 2001; Richter et al., 2002; Valdez, 1999; Woodard, 2002	9	0		0
1996 Stevens	Ciambrone, 1999; Russell & Smith, 1999; Stevens & Doerr, 1997	3	0		0
1996 Van Loon	Van Loon, 2000	1		Moneyham et al., 1996a	1
1996 Walker		0	0	Andrews et al., 1993; Frey, 1993	2
1997 Barnes et al.		0	0		0

(continued)

TABLE 3.1 Mutual Citations in Reports of Studies With HIV-Positive Women (Continued)

Reports	Who cited the author?	Number of Reports Cited	Whom did the authors cite?	Number of Reports Cited
1997 Bell	0	0	Frey, 1993 Salmon, 1993 Semple et al., 1993	3
1997 Bennett	0	0	Andrews et al. 1993 Coward, 1995 Hassin, 1994 Hutchison & Kurth, 1991 Moneyham et al., 1996a Rose, 1993 Semple et al., 1993 Weitz, 1993	8
1997 Demi et al.	Winstead et al., 2002	1	0	0
1997 Dozier	0	0	Weitz, 1993	1
1997 Faithfull	Marcenko & Samost, 1999 Tangenberg, 1998 Walsh, 2000	3	Andrews et al., 1993 Faithfull, 1992	2
1997 Gielen et al.	Schrimshaw et al., 2002	1	Hackl et al., 1997	1
1997 Grove et al.	Berger, 1998 Stanley, 1999	2	0	0
1997 Guillory et al.	Crane et al., 2000 Van Loon, 2000	4	0	0

Year & Author				References
1997 Hackl et al.	0	7	0	Woodard, 2002; Woodard & Sowell, 2001; Cameron, 2001; Ciambrone, 1999, 2001; Gielen et al., 1997; Marcenko & Samost, 1999; Van Loon, 2000; Winstead et al., 2002
1997 Leenerts	5	0	0	0; Andrews et al., 1993; Coward, 1995; Hutchison & Kurth, 1991; Rose, 1993; Sowell et al., 1997
1997 Siegel & Gorey	0	3	0	Cameron, 2001; Siegel, Lekas et al., 2001; Siegel & Schrimshaw, 2001
1997 Smith & Russell	0	1	0	Murdaugh et al., 2000
1997 Sowell & Misener	0	4		Leenerts, 1998; Leenerts & Magilvy, 2000; Misener & Sowell, 1998; Siegel & Schrimshaw, 2001
1997 Sowell et al.	0	4	0	Leenerts, 1997, 1998; Leenerts & Magilvy, 2000; Woodard & Sowell, 2001

(continued)

TABLE 3.1 Mutual Citations in Reports of Studies With HIV-Positive Women *(Continued)*

Reports	Who cited the author?	Number of Reports Cited	Whom did the authors cite?	Number of Reports Cited
1997 Stevens & Doerr	Ciambrone, 1999 Winstead et al., 2002	2	Hassin, 1994 Stevens, 1996	2
1998 Bedimo et al.	Siegel & Schrimshaw, 2001	1	0	0
1998 Berger	0	0	Grove et al., 1997	1
1998 Caba	0	0	0	0
1998 DeMarco et al.	Leenerts & Magilvy, 2000 Van Loon, 2000	2	Coward, 1995	1
1998 Dunbar et al.	Ciambrone, 1999 Goggin et al., 2001 Tangenberg, 1998, 2000, 2001 Van Loon, 2000	6	Regan-Kubinski & Sharts-Hopko , 1995 Seals et al., 1995 Semple et al., 1993	3
1998 Knight	0	0	0	0
1998 Leenerts	Bunting & Seaton, 1999	1	Moneyham et al., 1996a, b Seals et al., 1995 Sowell et al., 1996 Sowell et al., 1997 Sowell & Misener, 1997	6
1998 Misener & Sowell	Richter et al., 2002 Siegel, Lekas et al., 2001	2	Seals et al., 1995 Sowell et al., 1996 Sowell et al., 1997	3

1998 Raveis et al.	Valdez, 1999, 2001	2	0	0
1998 Serovich et al.	Schrimshaw et al., 2002	1	Kimberly et al., 1995	1
1998 Siegel et al.	0	0	0	0
1998 Stevens & Richards	Leenerts & Magilvy, 2000	1	0	0
1998 Tangenberg	0	0	Dunbar et al., 1998 Faithfull, 1997	2
1998 Van Servellen et al.	Van Loon, 2000	1	Semple et al., 1993	1
1998 Walker	Van Loon, 2000	1	Andrews et al., 1993 Frey, 1993	2
1999 Bunting & Seaton	Leenerts & Magilvy, 2000	1	Andrews et al., 1993 Leenerts, 1998 Moneyham et al., 1996a Sowell et al., 1996	4
1999 Chin & Kroesen	0	0	0	0
1999 Ciambrone	0	0	Dunbar et al., 1998 Hackl et al., 1997 Litwak et al., 1995 Moneyham et al., 1996a Seals et al., 1995 Semple et al., 1993 Stevens, 1996 Weitz, 1993	8

(continued)

TABLE 3.1 Mutual Citations in Reports of Studies With HIV-Positive Women (Continued)

Reports	Who cited the author?	Number of Reports Cited	Whom did the authors cite?	Number of Reports Cited
1999 Gray	0	0	Andrews et al., 1993	1
1999a Ingram & Hutchinson	Ingram & Hutchinson, 1999b; Santacroce et al., 2002	2	Andrews et al., 1993; Hutchison & Kurth, 1991; Ingram & Hutchinson, 1999b; Moneyham et al., 1996a; Rose, 1993	5
1999b Ingram & Hutchinson	Black & Miles, 2002; Ingram & Hutchinson, 1999a; Santacroce et al., 2002	3	Ingram & Hutchinson, 1999a; Moneyham et al., 1996a	2
1999 Leenerts	0	0	Leenerts, 1998	1
1999 Leenerts et al.	0	0	Leenerts, 1998, 1999; Sowell et al., 1996	3
1999 Marcenko & Samost	Schrimshaw et al., 2002; Tangenberg, 2000, 2001; Van Loon, 2000	4	Faithfull, 1997; Hackl et al., 1997; Weitz, 1993	3
1999 Russell & Smith	0	0	Andrews et al., 1993; Regan-Kubinski & Sharts-Hopko, 1995; Rose, 1993; Seals et al., 1995	6

Study				
1999 Stanley	0		Semple et al., 1993; Stevens, 1996	3
1999 Valdez	0		Grove et al., 1997; Hassin, 1994; Moneyham et al., 1996b; Moneyham et al., 1996a; Raveis et al., 1998; Seals et al., 1995; Sowell et al., 1996	4
2000 Crane et al.	0	0	Guillory et al., 1997	1
2000 Goicoechea-Balbona et al.	0	0	0	0
2000 Ingram et al.	Schrimshaw et al., 2002	1	Andrews et al., 1993; Hutchison & Kurth, 1991; Rose, 1993	3
2000 Leenerts & Magilvy	0		Andrews et al., 1993; Coward, 1995; DeMarco et al., 1998; Leenerts 1998, 1999; Moneyham et al., 1996a, b; Rose, 1993; Seals et al., 1995; Sowell et al., 1996	13

(continued)

TABLE 3.1 Mutual Citations in Reports of Studies With HIV-Positive Women *(Continued)*

Reports	Who cited the author?	Number of Reports Cited	Whom did the authors cite?	Number of Reports Cited
2000 Leenerts & Magilvy *(cont'd)*			Sowell et al., 1997 Sowell & Misener, 1997 Stevens & Richards, 1998	
2000 Murdaugh et al.	0	0	Smith & Russell, 1997	1
2000 Napravnik et al.	0	0	Hutchison & Kurth, 1991	1
2000 Siegel et al.	0	0	0	0
2000 Tangenberg	0	0	Dunbar et al., 1998 Marcenko & Samost, 1999	2
2000 Van Loon	0	0	DeMarco et al., 1998 Dunbar et al., 1998 Guillory et al., 1997 Hackl et al., 1997 Marcenko & Samost, 1999 Moneyham et al., 1996a Regan-Kubinski & Sharts-Hopko, 1995 Van Loon, 1996 Van Servellen et al., 1998 Walker, 1998	10

2000	Walsh	0	0	Andrews et al., 1993 Arnold, 1994 Faithfull, 1997 Hutchison & Kurth, 1991 Moneyham et al., 1996a, b Salmon, 1993 Semple et al., 1993	8
2000	Wesley et al.	0	0	0	0
2000	Williamson	0	0	0	0
2001	Cameron	0	0	Hackl et al., 1997 Hassin, 1994 Siegel & Gorey, 1997 Siegel & Schrimshaw, 2000	4
2001	Ciambrone	Ciambrone, 2002	1	Hackl et al., 1997 Weitz, 1993	2
2001	Goggin et al.	0	0	Dunbar et al., 1998 Semple et al., 1993	2
2001	Morrow et al.	0	0	0	0
2001	Moser et al.	0	0	Coward, 1995 Moneyham et al., 1996b Sowell et al., 1996	3

(continued)

TABLE 3.1 Mutual Citations in Reports of Studies With HIV-Positive Women (*Continued*)

Reports	Who cited the author?	Number of Reports Cited	Whom did the authors cite?	Number of Reports Cited
2001 Siegel, Lekas et al.	Cameron, 2001 Siegel & Schrimshaw, 2001	2	Misener & Sowell , 1998 Siegel & Gorey, 1997 Siegel & Schrimshaw, 2001	3
2001 Siegel & Schrimshaw	Siegel, Lekas et al., 2001	1	Bedimo et al., 1998 Siegel & Gorey, 1997 Siegel et al., 2001 Sowell et al., 1997	4
2001 Tangenberg	0	0	Dunbar et al., 1998 Marcenko & Samost, 1999	2
2001 Valdez	0	0	Raveis et al., 1998	1
2001 Woodard & Sowell	0	0	Coward, 1995 Guillory et al., 1997 Sowell et al., 1997	3
2002 Black & Miles	0	0	Ingram & Hutchinson, 1999b Kimberly et al., 1995 Moneyham et al., 1996a	3

2002 Ciambrone	0	0	Andrews et al., 1993 Ciambrone, 2001	2
2002 Haile et al.	0	0	Coward, 1995	1
2002 Richter et al.	0	0	Misener & Sowell, 1998 Sowell et al., 1996	2
2002 Sankar et al.	0	0	0	0
2002 Santacroce et al.	0	0	Ingram & Hutchinson, 1999a, b	2
2002 Schrimshaw & Siegel	0	0	Faithfull, 1997 Gielen et al., 1997 Ingram & Hutchinson, 2000 Kimberly et al., 1995 Marcenko & Samost, 1999 Moneyham et al., 1996a Semple et al., 1993 Serovich et al., 1998	8
2002 Winstead et al.	0	0	Demi et al., 1997 Hackl et al., 1997 Kimberly et al., 1995 Semple et al., 1993 Stevens & Doerr, 1997	5

(continued)

TABLE 3.1 Mutual Citations in Reports of Studies With HIV-Positive Women (*Continued*)

Reports	Who cited the author?	Number of Reports Cited	Whom did the authors cite?	Number of Reports Cited
2002 Woodard	0	0	Guillory et al., 1997 Leenerts, 1998 Moneyham et al., 1996a, b Moser et al., 2001 Sowell et al., 1996 Sowell & Misener, 1997 Sowell et al., 1997 Raveis et al., 1998 Rose, 1993 Woodard & Sowell, 2001	11

TABLE 3.2 Electronic Databases Used in the Metasynthesis Project

1. Academic Search Elite
2. AIDS Information Online (AIDSLINE)
3. Anthropological Index Online
4. Anthropological Literature
5. Black Studies
6. Cumulative Index to Nursing and Allied Health Literature (CINAHL)
7. Digital Dissertations
8. Dissertation Abstracts Index (DAI)
9. Educational Resource Information Center (ERIC)
10. MEDLINE
11. PsycInfo
12. Public Affairs Information Service (PAIS)
13. PubMed
14. Social Science Abstracts (SocSci Abstracts)
15. Social Science Citation Index
16. Social Work Abstracts
17. Sociological Abstracts
18. Women's Resources International
19. Women's Studies

TABLE 3.3 Search Concepts for Qualitative Research Methods Used
in the Metasynthesis Project

1. Case study
2. Constant comparison analysis
3. Content analysis
4. Conversation analysis
5. Descriptive study
6. Discourse/discourse analysis
7. Ethnography
8. Exploratory
9. Field observation
10. Field study
11. Focus group
12. Grounded theory
13. Hermeneutic
14. Interview/interview study
15. Narrative/narrative analysis
16. Naturalistic inquiry
17. Participant observation
18. Phenomenology
19. Qualitative study/qualitative research
20. Semiotics/semiotic analysis
21. Thematic analysis

TABLE 3.4 CINAHL (1982–Present) Evidence-Based Filters for Qualitative Research (Long Version) Using Ovid Search System

1. Qualitative Studies/
2. Ethnographic Research/
3. Phenomenological Research/
4. Ethnonursing Research/
5. Grounded Theory/
6. exp Qualitative Validity/
7. Purposive Sample/
8. exp Observational Methods/
9. Content Analysis/ or Thematic Analysis/
10. Constant Comparative Method/
11. Field Studies/
12. Theoretical Sample/
13. Discourse Analysis/
14. Focus Groups/
15. Phenomenology/ or Ethnography/ or Ethnological Research/
16. or/1-15
17. (qualitative or ethnon$ or phenomenol$).tw.
18. (grounded adj [theor$ or study or studies or research]).tw.
19. (constant adj [comparative or comparison]).tw.
20. (purpos$ adj sampl$4).tw.
21. (focus adj group$).tw.
22. (emic or etic or hermeneutic$ or heuristic or semiotics).tw.
23. (data adj1 saturat$).tw.
24. (participant adj observ$).tw.
25. (heidegger$ or colaizzi$ or spiegelberg$).tw.
26. (van adj manen$).tw.
27. (van adj kaam$).tw.
28. (merleau adj ponty$).tw.
29. (husserl$ or giorgi$).tw.
30. (field adj [study or studies or research]).tw.
31. lived experience$.tw.
32. narrative analysis.tw.
33. (discourse$3 adj analysis).tw.
34. human science.tw.
35. Life Experiences/
36. exp Cluster Sample/
37. or/1-36

Note: This filter was developed by the late Kathryn Nesbit, Database Education Specialist, Edward G. Miner Library, University of Rochester Medical Center, and is reproduced with the permission of the library. See http://www.urmc.rochester.edu/hslt/miner/digital_library/tip_sheets/Cinahl_eb_filters.pdf

REFERENCES

Barbour, R. S., & Barbour, M. (2003). Evaluating and synthesizing qualitative research: The need to develop a distinctive approach. *Journal of Evaluation in Clinical Practice, 9,* 179–186.

Bates, M. J. (1989). The design of browsing and berrypicking techniques for online search interface. *Online Review, 13,* 407–424.

Campbell, R., Pound, P., Pope, C., Britten, N., Pill, R., Morgan, M., et al. (2003). Evaluating meta-ethnography: A synthesis of qualitative research on lay experiences of diabetes and diabetes care. *Social Science & Medicine, 56,* 671–684.

Coletti, M. H., & Bleich, H. L. (2001). Medical subject headings used to search biomedical literature. *Journal of the American Medical Informatics Association, 8,* 317–323.

Cooper, H. (1998). *Synthesizing research: A guide for literature reviews* (3rd ed.). Thousand Oaks, CA: Sage.

Evans, D. (2002). Database searches for qualitative research. *Journal of the Medical Library Association, 90,* 290–293.

Gephart, R. P. (1988). *Ethnostatistics: Qualitative foundations for quantitative research.* Beverly Hills, CA: Sage.

Grant, M. J. (2004). How does your searching grow? A survey of search preferences and the use of optimal search strategies in the identification of qualitative research. *Health Information and Libraries Journal, 21,* 21–32.

Harris, M. R. (2005). The librarian's roles in the systematic review process: A case study. *Journal of the Medical Library Association, 93,* 81–87.

Harris, R. L. (1999). *Information graphics: A comprehensive illustrated reference.* New York: Oxford University Press.

Jasco, P. (1996). Ovid web gateway: Nobody does it better. *Online, 20(6),* 24–30.

Jones, M. L. (2004). Application of systematic review methods to qualitative research: Practical issues. *Journal of Advanced Nursing, 48,* 271–278.

Littleton, D., Marsalis, S., & Bliss, D. Z. (2004). Searching literature by design. *Western Journal of Nursing Research, 26,* 891–908.

Losee, R. M. (2000). When information retrieval measures agree about the relative quality of document rankings. *Journal of the American Society for Information Science, 51,* 834–840.

Marchionini, G. (1995). *Information seeking in electronic environments.* New York: Cambridge University Press.

Mason, J. (1996). *Qualitative researching.* London: Sage.

Meadow, C. T., Boyce, B. R., & Kraft, D. H. (2000). *Text information retrieval systems.* San Diego, CA: Academic Press.

Metz, M. H. (2000). Sociology and qualitative methodologies in educational research. *Harvard Educational Review, 70,* 60–74.

Morales, M. (1995). Uses of qualitative/quantitative terms in social and educational research. *Quality & Quantity, 29,* 39–53.

Nurius, P. S., & Yeaton, W. H. (1987). Research synthesis reviews: An illustrated critique of "hidden" judgments, choices, and compromises. *Clinical Psychology Review, 7,* 695–714.

Pound, P., Britten, N., Morgan, M., Yardley, L., Pope, C., Daker-White, G., et al. (2005). Resisting medicines: A synthesis of qualitative studies of medicine taking. *Social Science & Medicine, 61,* 133–155.

Sandelowski, M. (2003a). Qualitative research. In M. Lewis-Beck, A. E. Bryman, & T. F. Liao (Eds.), *The Sage encyclopedia of social science research methods* (Vol. 3, pp. 893–894). Thousand Oaks, CA: Sage.

Sandelowski, M. (2003b). Tables or tableaux? Writing and reading mixed methods studies. In A. Tashakkori & C. Teddlie (Eds.), *Handbook of mixed methods in social and behavioral research* (pp. 321–350). Thousand Oaks, CA: Sage.

Swanborn, P. G. (1996). A common base for quality control criteria in quantitative and qualitative research. *Quality & Quantity, 30,* 19–35.

Valsiner, J. (2000). Data as representations: Contextualizing qualitative and quantitative research strategies. *Social Science Information, 39,* 99–113.

Van Manen, M. (1990). *Researching lived experience: Human science for an action sensitive pedagogy.* Albany: State University of New York.

CHAPTER FOUR

Appraising Reports of Qualitative Studies

As you enter research reports into your synthesis study, you will begin to appraise each one. You will conduct both individual (intrareport) and comparative (interreport) appraisals.

INDIVIDUAL APPRAISAL

The purposes of individual appraisal are to: (a) determine whether reports meet your inclusion criteria; (b) ensure that your inclusion criteria require no further modification; and (c) familiarize yourself with the informational content, methodological orientation, style, and form of each report. Appraisal consists of appreciation and evaluation. The judgment that research findings are scientifically credible or relevant for practice (i.e., evaluation) can only be made after full understanding of the research reports containing these findings (i.e., appreciation). The full appreciation of qualitative research reports is achieved by connoisseurs of qualitative inquiry, or those individuals having a broad and deep understanding of its diversity and holding pluralist (as opposed to purist) views of its implementation (Johnson, Long, & White, 2001).

The reading guide that follows (see Box 4.1) will assist you to conduct judicious appraisals of qualitative research reports. You can read more about the intellectual context for and history of this guide in Sandelowski & Barroso (2002). We designed this guide for use with qualitative studies reported in the experimental/APA style (Bazerman, 1988), the preferred style of reporting the results of scientific inquiry. Other presentation styles (e.g., poems, novels, dramas, or deliberately anti-experimental/APA styles) do not have findings, or explicit databased interpretations offered by researchers, which can be integrated with other findings. Although important in their own right as art or as "celebrations" of data (Atkinson & Delamont, 2005, p. 823), these alternative presentations of qualitative research resist synthesis (often deliberately) and, thereby, have an equivocal place in qualitative research synthesis studies. (See Richardson, 2000, for an overview of such forms and Sandelowski, 2004, for a critique of such forms for the practice disciplines.)

The experimental/APA style of reporting research is a "prescriptive rhetoric" (Bazerman, 1988, p. 275) for reporting research that conceives the write-up as an objective description of a clearly defined and sequentially arranged process of inquiry, beginning with the identification of a research problem, and research questions or hypotheses, progressing through the selection of a sample and the collection of data, and ending with the analysis and transformation of those data into findings with implications for research and practice (Golden-Biddle & Lock, 1993; Gusfield, 1976). In these reports, content is presented in the third person passive voice and in defined introduction, review of literature, method, results, and discussion sections. In amended-experimental reports, content may be presented in the first person active voice and/or the results may be foreshadowed in the statement of the research purpose or, more typically, are merged with discussion of these results. The standardization of form evident in the experimental/APA report does not so much reflect the actual procedures of any particular study as it reinforces and reproduces the realist ideals and objectivist values associated with neo-positivist inquiry. Although this standardization of form is adhered to because of the belief that form ought not to confound content, form is inescapably content. Researchers/writers are expected to report their studies as if the in vivo execution of these studies conformed to the prescribed form for reporting them. They are expected to make real life conform to the page.

The purpose of the reading guide is to make more visible information you will likely want to have, but which amendments to the experimental style of reporting of information may make difficult to see. Sometimes the information you are seeking is there in a report, but it may not be located where you are looking for it, or be identified by researchers as that information. The guide helps you identify what you want to find in a research report, no matter where it is located or how it is presented and, thereby, enables you to appraise the report accurately and fairly.

You will see that the guide separates and orders the components constituting the typical empirical research report. This order will not necessarily be the order of the research report itself. You will also see that some categories of information cannot be fully appraised until the entire report is read, while other categories of information may be wholly contained in defined sections of a report. Any one statement from a research report may carry information applicable to more than one category, even though the writer of the report may have presented it as applicable to only one of them. For example, you may see a statement about how a researcher coded data as offering information that ought to be placed in both the data management and validity sections of the guide, even though the researcher never explicitly discussed coding in the context of validity or demonstrably conceived it as having anything to do with validity.

The guide also asks you to consider the presence or absence of information, and the relevance of that information, to your evaluation of the report. You may judge that a category of information has been addressed—either well or poorly—or has not been addressed at all, but decide that no matter whether or how it is addressed, it does not matter to you anyway in judging the overall value of the report. A report of a demonstrably ethnographic study may have little explicit description of method, but you can see method in the presentation of findings and, for that reason, judge this deficiency as minor, or not as a deficiency at all. Whether and how methods are described are functions of disciplinary norms and journal conventions. For example, reports in nursing and medical journals tend to give at least as much space to methods as to findings, while reports in social science journals tend to emphasize findings over methods.

In summary, by functioning to offset reporting inadequacies and to promote readers' understanding of themselves as readers, the guide serves as a corrective to the "narrow methodologism" often shaping the evaluation of qualitative reports (Eakin & Mykhalovskiy, 2003, p. 191) and, thereby, enhances their value. The guide helps you see what is there, where it is, and what is not there in a report. Together with the classification of findings (which we discuss in chapter 5), the guide helps you not only read reports, but also read into and against reports and even rewrite them to maximize the value of the findings in those reports. In a larger literary sense, a text cannot come fully into being until it is read. Moreover, not only does writing depend on reading, but also on the "generosity of the reader" (Manguel, 1996, p. 179) who is willing to expend the effort to make research reports more comprehensible and usable. The guide helps you better understand your inclinations and preferences as a reader of qualitative research reports. This is important because your reading preferences and expectations for qualitative research reports are the most important factors shaping your appraisal of these reports. In appraising each report, you are also appraising yourself as a reader, and this process will contribute to the reflexivity that will be evident in the research integration report you will ultimately write.

Once you have completed your reading of a report, you will be ready to consider its overall strengths. Note the information you judge to be deficient, and whether the kinds and number of deficiencies are sufficient to lower your evaluation of the study reported. For example, although you might not care that the grounded theory method was inaccurately depicted in a report, another reviewer might find in this "error" sufficient grounds to question the results of the study. Consider the extent to which the "noise" in a study, or its methodological flaws, detracts from its "signal," or potential value of study findings for practice (Edwards, Elwyn, Hood, & Rollnick, 2000; Edwards, Russell, & Stott, 1998). Characterize the report as having either acceptable or questionable value, and specifically note the reasons for your judgment.

Finally, the guide is meant to be used systematically but dynamically in interaction with each research report, not as a set of rules to be slavishly followed. You should accommodate the guide to the reports in your sample, not force the reports to fit the guide. For example, you may decide to use the appraisal parameters listed for each category systematically to mark only those items of special significance to you that you will include in the reviewer summary at the end of the guide. Or, you may decide to use it as a quantitative measurement tool, marking the presence and relevance of each parameter listed for every report in your study. You might develop an evaluation system whereby these items are differentially weighted and scored to accommodate items about which you care most and least. If you do decide to use the appraisal parameters as a quantitative measurement tool, you will be obliged to maximize and conduct ongoing evaluations of its intrarater, interrater, and internal consistency reliability.

We recommend using a hard copy of the guide, along with both hard and scanned copies of research reports, from which actual text can be copied directly into the template shown below. In the case of dissertations and books, where the volume of pages makes complete scans inefficient enterprises, at least scan the findings and sample characteristics.

Table 4.1 shows the results of using the reading guide to conduct an initial appraisal. We recommend that you now visit the supplement to chapter 4 at http://www.unc.edu/~msandelo/handbook/site/chapter4.html for a more dynamic presentation of the use of this guide.

COMPARATIVE APPRAISAL

After you have completed the detailed initial appraisal of each report in your study, you will be able to finalize the inclusion and exclusion criteria for your study and, thereby, settle on the reports that will definitely be included. You will also be ready to conduct a comparative appraisal across reports. Comparative appraisals allow you to create cross-study summaries and displays of key elements in included reports and prepare you for integrating the findings in these reports.

Cross-Case Displays and Summaries

The major device enabling comparative appraisals is a data display showing the same key elements of information in each report together. Such displays make it easier for you to describe relevant features of reports in the write-ups of your study, recognize reports derived from common parent studies and samples, and discern trends or patterns that will help you explain or contextualize the findings in these reports. Tabular displays allow you to make meta-study inferences and, thereby, provide an interpretive context for your synthesis. For example, you may see and draw inferences from the fact that most of the reports in your sample were written by or for nurses, most of the participants were women in minority groups, the modal sample size in the studies reported is 12 participants, the most prevalent stated theoretical frame of reference is loss, or that the most prevalent stated methodological frame of reference is symbolic interactionism. Thorne and her colleagues have shown the value of drawing inferences concerning how chronic illness has been studied and presented in qualitative research reports (e.g., Thorne, Joachim, Paterson, & Canam, 2002; Thorne et al., 2002). Greenhalgh and colleagues (2005) have shown the value of examining research traditions, or "metanarratives," in a domain of research to assess their impact on, and explain ostensible inconsistencies in, findings.

Cross-study tabular displays helped us see that the primary topic in the research purpose and findings in the reports of the positive prenatal diagnosis studies we reviewed was pregnancy termination. As shown in Figure 4.1, most of these reports are focused primarily on women's and couples' experiences of pregnancy termination following positive fetal diagnosis, not their experiences with fetal diagnosis per se. The failure to recognize this would have resulted in an invalid attribution of participant responses to diagnosis (as opposed to termination) and, thus, in an invalid integration. Figure 4.1 also shows that the reports varied in their temporal focus, with the findings in several reports focused narrowly on the diagnostic period, while the findings in other reports focused broadly on the entire trajectory of experience from diagnosis through the long-term aftermath of pregnancy termination.

The display of reports in Table 4.2 is organized alphabetically by the first author's last name, but you may decide to create more than one table

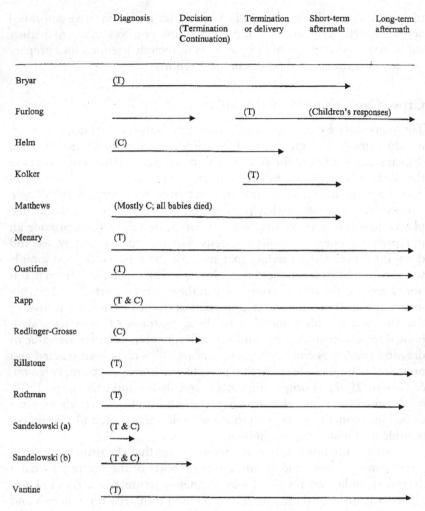

FIGURE 4.1 Comparison of topical and temporal focus of prenatal diagnosis reports.

with the same or different combinations of categories of information organized in more than one way (e.g., chronologically by year of publication, chronologically by years of data collection, by prevalence of topics of findings, by prevalence in sample size, or by any other organizing principle that is relevant to the purpose of your synthesis study). Playing with such displays during the course of your study allows you to interact with your data in different ways and, thereby, allows you to recognize patterns or trends you may not have noticed with only one display.

Items that tend to be included in data displays include sample size and configuration by sex, race/ethnicity, and age. But you will also want to include items directly relevant to the integration of findings you want to produce. For example, in our review of reports of studies with HIV-positive women, determining the stage and severity of disease at data collection was important to understanding women's reported experiences with the disease. In our review of studies with women or couples obtaining positive prenatal diagnoses, determining the types of prenatal tests and fetal diagnoses, and the timing of diagnoses, was important to understanding researchers' findings.

Data displays can be created using any word processing, data management, or data analysis system. Elements may be numerically coded for use with descriptive statistics. (We further address presentation styles and devices in chapter 9.)

Missing Information

Comparative appraisal also allows you to see what information is missing in individual reports relevant to producing a valid research integration of findings. You can make up for this lack of information by contacting the researchers who conducted the studies in question or, if this is not possible or researchers do not themselves have the missing information, by a variety of analytic techniques.

The part of research reports often missing relevant information is the sample section (Barroso & Sandelowski, 2003). In cases where no information is offered or available, you should indicate the numbers of reports that contain the category of information you are describing. For example, if you are describing the employment status of participants, you might write "in the 10 reports containing information on employment status, 15 women were employed and 30 women were unemployed," or show the varied Ns in a data display. You can also make up for reports that do not contain a category of information. For example, you can estimate the duration of disease in reports that do not explicitly present this information by determining the interval between year of diagnosis (which is reported) and one year prior to publication of the report, itself an estimate of when data collection ended. Accordingly, if a woman was reportedly diagnosed in 1993 and she appeared in a report published in 1998, the duration of disease can be assumed to be 4 years. If only a range of years of having a disease is provided, you can use the midpoint of the range to calculate the mean number of years since diagnosis and this can then be compared with other stated or calculated means.

In cases where information on the same topic (e.g., age of participants) is offered in diverse ways, you will want to make them comparable in order to summarize them. For example, whereas some researchers may state the numbers of participants in age intervals of 5, other researchers may actually give the ages of each participant or state only the range of ages for participants. You can compute weighted means (based on sample sizes) in order to make more comparable this diversity in reporting of age (Barroso & Sandelowski, 2003).

Comparing Findings

The most important target of comparative appraisal is the researchers' findings. You will ascertain the range and prevalence of topics. For example, among the topics addressed in the HIV reports were stigma, motherhood, living with HIV, and use of antiretroviral therapy. About 50% of the HIV reports we reviewed contained findings pertaining to motherhood, and about 80% findings pertaining to stigma and disclosure. In large sample research integration studies, the findings in each of these topical areas can become the focus of separate research integration projects, the findings of which can, in turn, be integrated.

Once findings have been grouped, you will then be able to determine whether they confirm, extend, refute, or complement each other. (We discuss the grouping of findings in chapter 6.)

Duplicate Reports

Comparative appraisal will also allow you to identify reports derived from common samples. Unless you pay close attention to sample characteristics, you may inadvertently overweight a finding contained in two or more reports from the same group of participants. The use of identical or overlapping samples in different research reports may not be readily evident as authors frequently do not refer to other reports derived from the same samples, including their own unpublished theses or dissertations. In addition, the same sample may be used by different investigators to conduct different analyses.

APPRAISAL AS FOUNDATION
FOR RESEARCH SYNTHESIS

The intra- and interreport appraisals you conduct are the foundation for your integration efforts. They constitute the data set you will use to integrate—while preserving the context for—findings. They must, therefore, be as accurate and considered as possible. (In chapter 8, we detail procedures for optimizing the descriptive and interpretive validity of study appraisals.)

BOX 4.1 Reading Guide for the Appraisal of Experimental/APA Style Qualitative Research Reports

Face Page

Create a basic inventory of the demographic features of and reading context for the research report, as shown below. Dating the study will help you evaluate the clinical relevance of findings. Findings may no longer be relevant, as when data from HIV-positive women were collected before the advent of antiretroviral therapy, when AIDS was considered a largely fatal as opposed to chronic disease. Such historical factors may cause you to alter your inclusion criteria for your integration study. After reviewing all of the reports in your sample, you will be able to ascertain which reports are related, or drawn from studies with the same or overlapping samples. This is important to preclude overweighting findings.

Demographic Features

Complete citation:
Author affiliations, including discipline and institution:
Funding source:
Acknowledgments:
Period of data collection:
Geographic location of study:
Dates of submission and acceptance of work:
Publication type (e.g., authored/edited book, journal, dissertation, thesis, conference proceeding):
Mode of retrieval (e.g., computer data base, citation list, personal communication):
Key words (as stated in report):
Abstract (copied from report):
Related reports (determined after appraisal of all reports):

Reading Context

Date of reading:
Reader:
Purpose of reading:
Reader affiliations:
Authored by reviewer, or member of review team (Y/N)?

Research Problem

Extract or paraphrase all statements concerning what the writer thinks is wrong, missing, or requires changing. The research problem is usually a clinical problem in the practice disciplines, and a theoretical or disciplinary problem in the social science disciplines. An example of a clinical or practice problem is:

> Many women with HIV wait too long to obtain treatment. Delays in obtaining HIV-related treatment have been linked to shorter survival for women after diagnosis. These delays must be stopped, but we do not know enough about why they occur.

An example of a theoretical problem is:

> Stigma has generally been conceived as a negative event. But there are circumstances in which stigma has positive outcomes. Theories of stigma should be expanded to include these positive outcomes.

Generally appearing early in (amended-)experimental style research reports, problem statements set the stage for the study that was conducted, or the results of the specific analysis reported, and they typically establish the significance of and/or reason for the research purpose and questions. Problems may be explicitly stated or they may be implied in the research purpose and/or the literature review.

Appraisal parameters	Presence/ Relevance +/−	+/−	Reviewer comments
1. There is a discernible problem that led to the study.			
2. The problem is accurately depicted.			
3. The problem is comprehensively depicted.			
4. The problem is related to the research purpose and/or the literature review.			
5. The description of the problem establishes the significance of the research purpose, or why the researcher wanted to conduct the study, beyond simply stating that "no one has studied this (qualitatively) before."			
6. The claim that "no one has studied this before" is accurate.			

Research Purpose(s) & Question(s)

Extract or paraphrase all statements concerning one or more immediate and long-term goals, objectives, or aims of the study, and/or a list of one or more questions the study findings will answer. Research purposes and questions generally appear early in (amended-)experimental reports. Purposes may be explicitly stated, or they may be apparent in statements such as "I intend/hope to show . . ." or "I will argue/suggest . . ." Statements of purpose may be found in the foreshadowing or summarizing of the research findings early in the report.

Because research purposes and questions may change as data collection and analysis proceed, the research purposes and questions described in a report may either be the ones that were originally conceived going into the field of study, or that were altered in the course of the study.

Appraisal parameters	Presence/ Relevance +/–	+/–	Reviewer comments
1. There is a discernible set of research purposes and/or questions.			
2. Research purposes or questions are linked to the research problem and/or to the review of literature.			
3. Research purposes and questions are amenable to qualitative study.			
4. Researchers clarify whether the research purposes and questions are those that preceded entry into the field of study or were altered in the course of study to accommodate data analysis.			

Literature Review

Extract or paraphrase researchers' discussion of what is believed, known, and not known about the research problem, and of how the problem has been studied. The literature review usually precedes the method section in (amended-) experimental style reports. Sometimes the literature reviewed is combined with information about the research problem, while at other times, it is set off in a separate section and labeled as a literature review, or with headers referring to topics or themes contained in the review. In addition, introductory reviews of literature in qualitative research reports may clarify the research problem that originally led to the study, or set the interpretive scene for the research findings that are the outcomes of the study.

Reviews of literature may show one or a combination of the following logics pointing toward the research purpose:

1. A *deficit/gap* logic whereby writers emphasize what is not known about a research problem and point to a research purpose that will offset this knowledge deficit;
2. An *error* logic whereby writers emphasize what is mistaken about what is presumably known about a research problem and point to a research purpose that will correct this error;
3. A *contradiction* logic whereby writers emphasize inconsistencies in knowledge about a research problem and point to a research purpose that will help to resolve this contradiction and/or;
4. A *linking* logic whereby writers emphasize the common areas in two or more seemingly disparate bodies of empirical, theoretical, or other literature related to the research problem and point to a research purpose that will address this overlap.

Appraisal parameters	Presence/ Relevance +/- +/-	Reviewer comments
1. Key studies and other relevant literatures addressing the research problem are included.		
2. The review addresses the research problem.		
3. The review clarifies whether it reflects what researchers knew and believed going into the field of study—before any data were collected—or came to know and believe while in or leaving the field of study, after data analysis began or was completed.		
4. The review shows a critical attitude toward the accumulated knowledge about the research problem and toward the methods used to study it, as opposed to indiscriminately identifying or summarizing studies in a *he said/she said* format.		
5. The review shows a discernible logic that points toward the research purpose, and is not at odds with it (e.g., as when researchers use a gap logic to criticize the prevalence of descriptive studies in an area and then report another descriptive study).		

Orientation Toward the Target Phenomenon

Extract or paraphrase all statements indicating the perspectives, assumptions, conceptual/theoretical frameworks, philosophies and/or other frames of reference, mindsets, "theoretical sensitivities," or orientations guiding or influencing researchers concerning the target phenomenon, or subject matter of a study (i.e., the people, events, or things to be studied), regardless of whether researchers appear to be aware of them. For example, Goffman's theory of stigma is used to frame a study of HIV-positive women's social interactions. Such frames of reference may be explicitly stated, as in the Goffman example. Or, they may be implied (and sometimes not recognized as an orientation) in the language used in the introductory sections of the research report, as when miscarriage is referred to as a "loss," HIV-positive women's responses to infection are discussed in terms of "self-care" or "coping," and studies in perinatal bereavement, self-care, or coping are reviewed. The orientation toward the target phenomenon may be clearly distinguishable from the orientation toward inquiry in a study, or may overlap with it. For example, feminism may be presented as the framework for the study of women's responses to HIV diagnosis, in particular, and/or as the framework for any study of women and/or for inquiry, in general. A frame of reference may have influenced a study from its conception through the interpretation of findings. Or, a frame of reference may not have entered the study until after some or all of the data were collected and analyzed. For example, Goffman's ideas about stigma may have been the a priori or sensitizing framework for a study of women with HIV. That is, these women were seen from the beginning through to the end of the study as living with and responding to a culturally stigmatizing condition. In contrast, Goffman's ideas might have entered a study only after researchers had begun to analyze their data and recognized that women's responses fit and/or were illuminated by these ideas.

Appraisal parameters	Presence/ Relevance +/− +/−	Reviewer comments
1. There is an explicitly stated or implied frame of reference.		
2. If explicitly stated, the frame of reference is accurately rendered.		
3. Whether stated or implied, the frame of reference fits the target phenomenon and is not forced onto it.		
4. If explicitly stated as the guiding frame of reference for a study, it played a discernible role in the way the study was conducted and/or the way the findings were treated. This is in contrast to a frame of reference that is evidently operating in a study, but that is not demonstrably recognized by the researcher (e.g., as when HIV-positive women are consistently referred to as being "in denial," but denial as a concept is never discussed or recognized for its interpretive heritage or impact. Or, when researchers do not recognize that they are viewing self-care as activities health care providers view as positive and not as encompassing such activities as smoking and drug abuse, which can also be construed as self-care).		
5. The presentation of the orientation of the study clarifies whether it influenced researchers going into the field of study—before any data were collected—or after data analysis began or was completed.		
6. The researchers demonstrate awareness of their orientations in their review or in their presentation or discussion of findings.		

Orientation Toward Inquiry

Extract or paraphrase all statements indicating the perspectives, assumptions, philosophies, methods, and/or other frames of reference guiding or influencing researchers concerning the conduct of a study. For example, grounded theory is presented as the method and as deriving from tenets of symbolic interactionism and pragmatism. Semiotics is presented as the analytic frame of reference for the study of a document or artifact. Such frames of reference may be explicitly stated, or implied in the method language and/or citations used. For example, no method may ever be named per se, but phrases such as "lived experience," suggesting phenomenology, and "theoretical sampling," suggesting grounded theory, are used; and/or there are citations to Van Manen's work on phenomenology or Strauss's & Corbin's work on grounded theory. The orientation toward inquiry may be clearly distinguishable from the orientation toward the target phenomenon of a study, or it may overlap with it. For example, social constructionism may be presented as the framework for any study of women and/or for inquiry, in general, and for a study of women's responses to HIV diagnosis, in particular.

Appraisal parameters	Presence/ Relevance +/– +/–	Reviewer comments
1. There is a stated or implied method.		
2. The method fits the research purpose.		
3. The method is accurately rendered.		
4. The method is appropriately used.		
5. The uses of method-linked techniques for other than method-linked purposes are explained (e.g., as when theoretical sampling is used in a qualitative descriptive study, or phenomenological techniques are used to create items for an instrument).		
6. Researchers demonstrate awareness of method choices and their impact on findings.		
7. The study is methodologically qualitative.		

Sampling Strategy & Techniques

Extract or paraphrase all information about researchers' sampling intentions going into a study and the sampling intentions and decisions that evolved in the course of the study, including the rationale for the recruitment sites selected.

Appraisal parameters	Presence/ Relevance +/– +/–	Reviewer comments
1. The sampling plan fits the research purpose and method.		

Appraisal parameters	Presence/ Relevance +/–	+/–	Reviewer comments

2. The sampling plan is purposeful, and the type(s) of purposeful sampling is/are specified.
3. The sampling plan described is accurately rendered, as opposed to being inaccurately rendered or misrepresented (e.g., as when maximum variation sampling is presented as having equal numbers of men and women, or percents of African Americans or Hispanic Americans equal to their presence in a population).
4. Sampling intentions going into a study are sufficiently differentiated from sampling intentions evolving in the course of study.
5. Sites of recruitment fit the research purpose and sampling strategy.

Sample Size & Composition

Extract or paraphrase all information concerning the people, places, events, documents, and/or artifacts comprising the actual sources of information for the study, and the actual sites from which people were recruited. Include here all descriptions of the sample, including the members of focus groups. Because ethnographic studies are typically site- or place-bound, *site* is actually a component of the sample. Site—as sample—is contrasted with site of data collection. That is, a study may involve one organization (site as sample), and interviews may be conducted in conference rooms on site (site of data collection).

Appraisal parameters	Presence/ Relevance +/–	+/–	Reviewer comments

1. Sample size and configuration fit the research purpose and sampling strategy.
2. Sample size and configuration can support claims to informational redundancy, or theoretical or scene saturation.
3. Sample size and configuration can support claims to the intensive and comprehensive study of particulars.
4. Sample size and configuration support the findings.

Appraisal parameters	Presence/ Relevance +/− +/−	Reviewer comments
5. Sample composition is accurately and appropriately displayed in variable- and/or case-oriented arrangements.		
6. Numbers are used appropriately to describe samples, as opposed to inappropriately used (e.g., as when a designation of "50% of the sample" refers to only two participants, or when only the mean or range is reported for participant ages that range from 18–70).		
7. Features of the sample critical to the understanding of findings are described, as opposed to not described (e.g., as when, in a study of HIV-positive women's reproductive decision making, no information is offered on women's use of contraceptives, obstetric histories, or on severity of disease).		
8. The number of and reason why eligible participants refused to participate or left the study are described.		
9. Sites of recruitment fit the evolving sampling needs of the study.		

Data Collection or Generation Techniques & Sources

Extract or paraphrase all information concerning sources of, or the techniques or procedures used to obtain or generate the data for, the study in the following categories: interviews (including focus groups), observations, documents, and artifacts. Extract or paraphrase descriptions of the: (a) purpose, place, and number per participant or event of interviews or observations; (b) type of, orientation to, and/or manner of conducting interviews, observations, document reviews, or artifact study; and (c) content, timing, and sequencing of data collection or generation. Extract or paraphrase information about alterations in techniques and procedures made in the course of the study.

Appraisal parameters	Presence/ Relevance +/–	+/–	Reviewer comments
1. Sources of data and techniques of data collection or generation fit the evolving needs of the study.			
2. The content, sequence, and timing of data collection or generation techniques fit the purpose and orientations of the study, as opposed to not fitting them (e.g., as when the purpose of a study is to ascertain structural barriers to health care utilization, but the only sources of data are women's perceptions of their health care providers. Or, researchers conflate the longitudinal with the validation purpose for conducting more than one interview with the same participants or more than one observation of the same event).			
3. Specific data collection or generation techniques were demonstrably tailored to the reported study, as opposed to the presentation of textbook or rote descriptions of data collection or generation with no application shown to the study reported.			
4. Data collection or generation techniques are accurately rendered, as opposed to inaccurately rendered (e.g., as when the observation of process that occurs during interviews and focus groups is presented as participant observation).			
5. The sources of data presented are demonstrably the basis of the findings, as opposed to not being their basis (e.g., as when document study is presented as a data collection strategy, but there is no evidence of its use).			
6. Data collection or generation techniques are correctly used, as opposed to misused (e.g., as when focus groups are conducted by asking each parti-cipant in turn to answer the same question, instead of posing a question to the group to stimulate group interaction.			
7. Sites are conducive to data collection or generation.			

Appraisal parameters	Presence/ Relevance +/− +/−	Reviewer comments
8. The time period for data collection or generation is explicitly stated.		
9. The timing of data collection or generation vis-à-vis the target events featured in the study is explicitly stated (e.g., interviews were conducted within 2 months of diagnosis).		
10. The timing of use of data collection or generation techniques vis-à-vis each other is explicitly stated (e.g. observations took place before the interviews).		

Data Management & Analysis Techniques

Extract or paraphrase descriptions of techniques or procedures used to: (a) create an audit trail of data; (b) prepare data for analysis; (c) catalog, file, or organize data; and (d) break up, (dis)play (with), and/or reconfigure data. Included here is information on whether and how transcripts of interviews and field notes were prepared, whether and which computerized text management systems were used, the specific analytic approaches employed (e.g., content, constant comparison, narrative, discourse, or other analysis), and whether and how coding schemes, data matrices, and other visual displays of data were used. Information about these techniques may be explicitly stated, illustrated, or evident in the findings.

Appraisal parameters	Presence/ Relevance +/− +/−	Reviewer comments
1. Data management & analysis techniques fit the research purposes and data.		
2. Specific data management & analysis techniques were tailored to the reported study, as opposed to textbook or rote descriptions of data management & analysis being offered, with no application shown to the study reported.		
3. Data management & analysis techniques are accurately rendered.		
4. Data management & analysis techniques are correctly used.		

Appraisal parameters	Presence/ Relevance +/– +/–	Reviewer comments
5. Analysis of data fits the data, as opposed to not fitting them (e.g., as when focus group data are analyzed at the individual level and the analysis takes no account of group interaction).		
6. There is a clear description of how different data sets were analytically linked.		

Orientation to and Techniques for Maximizing Validity

Extract or paraphrase information indicating views of, and techniques or procedures intended to optimize, scientific or ethnographic validity. Included here is information about the stated strengths and limitations of a study, and discussion of reflexivity, auditability, reliability, rigor, credibility, and plausibility, and of specific procedures implemented, such as member validation and peer review. Information about validity may be explicitly stated or implied in discussions of sampling, data collection and analysis, and in the presentation of the findings. Researchers may offer information about, but not necessarily identify or even recognize in this information, different kinds of validation approaches (e.g., interview techniques, coding schemes) or validities (e.g., descriptive, interpretive, theoretical, and pragmatic validity).

Appraisal parameters	Presence/ Relevance +/– +/–	Reviewer comments
1. Researchers show an awareness of their influence on the study and its participants.		
2. The distinctive limitations of the study are appropriately summarized (e.g., theoretical sampling could not be fully conducted in a grounded theory study), as opposed to inappropriately summarized (e.g., as when researchers apologize for the so-called limitations of qualitative research).		
3. Techniques for validation are used that fit the purpose, method, sample, data, and findings, as opposed to using techniques that do not fit (e.g., as when reliability coding to ascertain consistency in interview data is used in a study emphasizing the revisionist nature of narratives).		

Appraisal parameters	Presence/ Relevance +/- +/-	Reviewer comments
4. Techniques used are tailored to the reported study, as opposed to presentations of textbook or rote descriptions of validation techniques with no application shown to the study reported.		
5. Techniques for validation are accurately rendered, as opposed to misrepresented (e.g., as when interpretive validity, the actor's point of view, is confused with theoretical validity, or the researcher's interpretation, and triangulation for convergent validity is confused with using different data sources for informational completeness or to obtain multiple perspectives).		
6. Techniques for validation are correctly used, as opposed to incorrectly used (e.g., as when cases are kept in or dropped from consideration because they conform or do not conform to other cases).		

Findings

Extract or paraphrase statements of what researchers "found" from the data they collected, or the results or interpretation of these data. In (amended-) experimental reports, a finding is a data-based discovery, conclusion, judgment, pronouncement, or interpretation researchers offer about the events, experiences, or cases under investigation. In these reports, findings are generally distinguishable from: (a) data, or the case descriptions, field notes, quotations, or other empirical material researchers offer in support of their interpretations; (b) analysis, or the data management, coding, and other data amplification, complication, and reduction techniques researchers used to create their interpretations; and from (c) researchers' efforts to signify or translate findings for future research, practice, or policy. The finding in a grounded theory study is the theory, the finding in an ethnographic study is the ethnography, and the finding in a phenomenologic study is the phenomenology. In experimental-style reports, findings are located in the results section. In amended-experimental reports, they may also be located in the discussion section, or foreshadowed in the introduction to the report.

Appraisal parameters	Presence/ Relevance +/– +/–	Reviewer comments
1. The report contains findings, as opposed to having no findings (e.g., as when data are presented with virtually no interpretation of them).		
2. Findings are distinguishable from other elements of the research report.		
3. Interpretations of data are demonstrably plausible and/or sufficiently substantiated with data collected for or generated in the study reported.		
4. Data are sufficiently (i.e., neither over- nor under-) analyzed and interpreted.		
5. Findings address the ultimate purpose of the study reported, as opposed to not addressing it (e.g., as when the stated purpose of a study was to describe structural barriers to health care utilization, but the findings focus on women's perceptions of their health care).		
6. Variations in findings by relevant sample characteristics are addressed.		
7. Variations in findings by time (in event and research trajectory) are addressed.		
8. Analysis is largely case-oriented, or oriented to the study of particulars, as opposed to variable-oriented, or quantitatively informed.		
9. Quantitative transformations of data are demonstrably in the service of qualitative interpretation.		
10. Ideas (e.g., concepts, themes) are precise, well developed, and linked to each other.		
11. The results offer new information about, insight into, or a reformulation of the target phenomenon.		

Discussion & Implications

Extract or paraphrase statements summarizing or drawing conclusions about the findings of the study, and indicating their transferability and clinical, theoretical, policy, disciplinary, or other significance. In experimental-style reports, this information appears at the end. In amended-experimental reports, the signification of findings or comparison of findings to findings in other studies often appears in the results section.

Appraisal parameters	Presence/ Relevance +/− +/−	Reviewer comments
1. Discussion of findings is based on the findings presented, as opposed to being contrary to the findings or introducing new findings.		
2. Findings are linked to findings in other studies or to other relevant literatures either previously discussed or newly introduced.		
3. The clinical, policy, theoretical, disciplinary, and/or other significance of the findings is thoughtfully considered, as opposed to indiscriminately considered (e.g., as when changes in practice are recommended that merely propose actions opposite to the findings [providers are found to be insensitive so the implication is that they must be educated to become sensitive], or when repeating a study with other populations and/or in other settings is recommended with no rationale).		
4. The location and extent to which the findings are transferable are clarified.		

Protection of Human Subjects

Extract or paraphrase descriptions of issues and practices relating to the recruitment, retention, and well-being of the human participants in a study. Included here is information concerning how participants were approached and enrolled in the study, the informed consent procedures used, the benefits and risks participants were subjected to by virtue of being in the study, the inducements and protections offered them, and the way they responded to participation in the study.

Appraisal parameters	Presence/ Relevance +/–	+/–	Reviewer comments
1. Benefits and risks distinctive to the study reported are addressed, as opposed to textbook or rote descriptions of human subjects issues being offered with no discussion of their particular relevance to the reported study.			
2. Recruitment and consent techniques were tailored to fit the sensitivity of the subject matter and/or vulnerability of participants.			
3. Data collection and management techniques were tailored to fit the sensitivity of the subject matter and/or vulnerability of participants.			
4. Examples of data provided as evidence to support findings have analytical value and present participants fairly, as opposed to having only sensational value or presenting participants unfairly (e.g., as when extreme incidents of events are presented when others would do, or when quotes are edited to emphasize the lack of education of certain participants when this is not analytically relevant).			

Logic & Form of Findings

Instead of extracting or paraphrasing the informational contents of reports, here you are concentrating on the presentational logic and form of the findings, including the literary and visual devices used to present the study and its findings. Consider such features as language expression (e.g., metaphors or controlling images) in the title of the report and its sections, and in the way findings are organized and presented. Consider the uses of quotations, numbers, vignettes, and visual displays (e.g., tables, figures, diagrams, photos).

Qualitative findings may be presented according to one or more of the following presentation logics:

1. quantitatively and thematically, by most to least prevalent or most to least important theme;
2. temporally and thematically, with the clock time of the research participants as the primary organizing principle and theme as the secondary organizing principle;
3. thematically and temporally, with theme as the primary organizing principle and the clock time of the participants as the secondary organizing principle;
4. narratively, as a day/week/month/year in the life of participants;

5. narratively, as an unfolding tragedy, comedy, or melodrama in the life of participants;
6. perspectivally (Rashômon effect), by manifestly juxtaposing different points of view of participants and/or of researchers;
7. polyvocally, by manifestly juxtaposing different voices of participants and/or of researchers;
8. conceptually, by using sensitizing concepts from extant theory;
9. conceptually, by using a grounded theory template for analysis, such as the conditional matrix, typology, or transition format, or set of working hypotheses;
10. episodically, emphasizing key moments of an experience;
11. archaeologically, with the clock time of researchers as the primary organizing principle to show how the understanding of an event unfolded for them; and/or
12. via representative, exemplary, and/or composite cases or vignettes.

Classify the findings (see chapter 5) as either surveys or syntheses of the data researchers collected or generated in a study, or as having no findings.

1. No finding (exclude from integration study)
2. Surveys
   a. Topical surveys
   b. Thematic surveys
3. Syntheses
   a. Conceptual or thematic descriptions
   b. Interpretive explanations

Appraisal parameters	Presence/ Relevance +/－ +/－	Reviewer comments
1. The overall presentation of the study fits its purpose, method, and findings.		
2. Given the reporting style, elements of the research report are placed where readers are likely to find them.		
3. Data are transformed into findings.		
4. There is a coherent logic to the presentation of findings.		
5. Findings are organized in ways that do analytic justice to them, as opposed to not doing them justice (e.g., as when, in a rendering of women's experiences with HIV as having physical, psychosocial, and spiritual aspects, highly disparate ideas are dumped into each section because, on the surface, they share physical, psychosocial, and spiritual features).		

Appraisal parameters	Presence/ Relevance +/– +/–	Reviewer comments

6. Visual displays, quotations, cases, and numbers clarify, summarize, substantiate, or otherwise illuminate the findings, as opposed to being at odds with them (e.g., as when a quotation has more ideas in it than featured by the researcher, or a path diagram shows a relationship between variables at odds with the relationship between them depicted in the text).

7. The numerical meaning of such terms as "most," "some," "sometimes," and "commonly" is clear.

8. The empirical referent for a theme or concept is clear, as opposed to theme or concept being conflated with experience (e.g., as when a researcher states that five themes emerged from the data instead of stating that women managed their symptoms in one of five ways. Or, the writer does not clarify whether the themes discussed are strategies to accomplish a goal, outcomes of having engaged in these strategies, typologies of behavior, or milestones and turning points in a transition).

9. Findings are presented in a comparative and parallel fashion, as opposed to a noncomparative or nonparallel manner (e.g., as when, in a typology, some types are presented as behaviors, while others are presented as character traits, and each type is not compared to every other type).

10. Quotations are appropriately staged, as opposed to inappropriately staged (e.g., as when only "one woman said" and "another woman said" lead into quotations).

11. Titles of paper and section headers reflect their contents.

12. The overall presentation of the study is audience-appropriate.

Reviewer's Abstract & Summary Appraisal

In this section, annotate the key features of the report as you see them without regard to what writers claimed for them. Here you are documenting the logic-in-use, as opposed to the reconstructed logic of the study. The varied use of methods, and words to designate them, makes it essential to determine what was actually done in a study—to the extent that this can be ascertained from the report of the study—rather than depending on researchers' own characterizations of what they did. If no information is explicitly offered in a category, state "not specified," and then state what you consider to characterize the study in that category. Give the key sample characteristics most relevant to understanding the findings (e.g., primarily minority women of childbearing age with nonsymptomatic HIV infection). Extract the key findings of the report and edit them both to stay close to the findings as presented in the report, and to remain clear to all readers, regardless of whether they have read the report. Use the specific appraisal parameters in any consistent way you see fit to judge the overall value of the study as acceptable or questionable.

Research purpose:
Theoretical framework:
Method:
Sample size & key characteristics
Data collection techniques:
Data analysis techniques:
Primary topic of findings:
Secondary topics of findings:

Type of findings (see chapter 5):   No finding (exclude from study)____
                                    Topical survey____
                                    Thematic survey____
                                    Conceptual/thematic description____
                                    Interpretive explanation____

Extracted & edited findings (see chapter 6):

Evaluation: Acceptable (Signal > noise)____
              Questionable (Noise > signal)____

Summary comments:

TABLE 4.1 Use of Reading Guide to Conduct an Initial Appraisal of a Research Report

[Face Page]

Complete citation: Siegel, K., & Schrimshaw, E. W. (2001). Reasons and justifications for considering pregnancy among women living with HIV/AIDS. *Psychology of Women Quarterly, 25,* 112–123.

Author affiliations: Public health & psychology, Columbia University

Funding source: None stated

Acknowledgments: None stated

Period of data collection: January 1996 to April 1997

Geographic location of study: New York City

Date of submission: February 7, 2000

Date of acceptance: Initial acceptance, June 15, 2000; Final acceptance, November 17, 2000

Publication type: Women's journal

Mode of retrieval: E Database

Key words: None

Abstract (copy block from article): Despite the risks associated with pregnancy, available data suggest that HIV-infected women are no less likely to become pregnant than uninfected women. To understand HIV-infected women's reasons for wanting to have a child, focused interviews were conducted with a predominantly minority sample of 51 HIV-infected women in New York City. They were noted to actively weigh both the potential risks and benefits of their pregnancy decisions. Women reported three major reasons for wanting a child: (1) her husband/boyfriend really wants children, (2) having missed out on raising her other children, and (3) believing that a child would make her feel complete, fulfilled, and happy. Women also reported several justifications that they believed offset the risks of pregnancy, including: (1) other HIV-infected women were having healthy babies, (2) feeling optimistic about having a healthy baby due to the prophylactic effects of AZT (zidovudine), (3) having faith that God will protect the child, (4) being young and "healthy" will prevent transmission, and (5) feeling that she is better able to raise a child now. These findings suggest that to make fully informed pregnancy decisions, women should be encouraged to explore their reasons for wanting pregnancy, as well as discuss the potential risks.

Related reports: Siegel, K., Lekas, H. M., Schrimshaw, E. W., & Johnson, J. K. (2001). Factors associated with HIV-infected women's use or intention to use AZT during pregnancy. *AIDS Education and Prevention, 13,* 189–206.

Date of review: 11/27/01

Reviewer: MS

Purpose of review: Initial appraisal

Authored by reviewer, or member of review team? No

(continued)

TABLE 4.1 Use of Reading Guide to Conduct an Initial Appraisal of a Research Report *(Continued)*

Research problem	As we enter the third decade of the HIV/AIDS epidemic, women have become one of the fastest growing populations living with the disease in the United States (Centers for Disease Control [CDC], 1999). The cumulative number of reported AIDS cases among women has risen dramatically in recent years, from 44,000 in 1993 (CDC, 1994a) to nearly 120,000 by the end of 1999 (CDC, 1999). Further, women account for 23% of all new AIDS cases and 32% of all new HIV infections reported in 1999 (CDC, 1999). About 80% of women with AIDS are 13–44 years of age—within their prime reproductive years. It has been estimated that approximately 7,000 infants are born to HIV-infected women each year; of these 1,000 to 2,000 will be HIV infected (Davis, Byers, Lindgren, Caldwell, Karon, & Gwinn, 1995). Yet, despite the increasing prevalence of women living with HIV/AIDS, little research has addressed their attitudes and concerns about childbearing.

Few studies have investigated the factors that influence reproductive decisions of HIV-infected women.

To date, there has been little research into the reasons infected women may desire a child. |
| Research purpose(s)/ question(s) | *Many might view HIV-infected women as selfish or deviant for desiring a child or becoming pregnant. Because of this, it is especially important to give voice to these women's own reasons and justifications for their pregnancy. Further, an understanding of the reasons they offer for wanting pregnancy are crucial to gaining insight into the reproductive desires and decisions of HIV-infected women.* The present study extends work in this area by investigating not only the reasons women offered for their desire to become pregnant, but also the beliefs these women used to justify these desires. |
| Literature review | Risks of HIV and Pregnancy

Given the possible risks associated with pregnancy and childbearing while HIV infected, young women living with HIV/AIDS face difficult reproductive decisions. One significant risk is the transmission of infection to the newborn. Fortunately, when the antiviral drug AZT (zidovudine) is taken on a specific regimen by the mother during the course of the pregnancy and by the infant following birth, it has been found to lower transmission rates to approximately 8% of all births to infected mothers, compared to 25% if untreated (CDC, 1994b; Connor, Sperling, Gelber, Kiselev, Scott, |

TABLE 4.1 *(Continued)*

O'Sullivan, VanDyke, Bey, Shearer, Jacobson, Jimenez, O'Neill, Bazin, Delfraissy, Culnane, Coombs, Elkins, Moye, Stratton, & Balsley, 1994). Although newer, more effective treatments for infected individuals are now widely used, their utility in preventing perinatal transmission remains under investigation, and AZT continues to be the recommended treatment for HIV-infected pregnant women (CDC, 1998). This new avenue for the primary prevention of perinatal transmission is a significant and welcomed development; however, it is unclear whether sufficiently early initiation of AZT or adequate adherence to the prescribed regimen (for both mother and infant) is typically achieved outside the structured environment of a clinical trial. Among pregnant, infected women, delays in initiating treatment and nonadherence may occur as a result of the pervasive negative attitudes toward AZT (e.g., AZT is toxic and does more harm than good) and its side effects (Siegel & Gorey, 1997; Siegel, Lekas, Schrimshaw, & Johnson, in press).

An additional reproductive concern for women living with HIV/AIDS is the risk that an uninfected, prospective, biological father will become infected while attempting conception. Although this risk can be obviated through artificial insemination, it is unclear if this would be an affordable or acceptable procedure to most socioeconomically disadvantaged women or couples. When the prospective father is already infected, the risk of possible reinfection with another strain of the virus may also be a concern for both the man and the woman. Infected women considering pregnancy may also worry about the potential negative impact on their own health from the physiological and psychological stresses of pregnancy, although the validity of such concerns remains unclear (Landers, Martinez, & Coyne, 1997). Finally, uncertainty regarding their future health and ability to fulfill the responsibilities of motherhood may also be a concern for infected women contemplating pregnancy.

Despite these acknowledged risks and concerns, research suggests that many HIV-infected women apparently maintain a strong desire to have children. Extant research on the incidence of pregnancy among seropositive women when compared with uninfected women suggests that HIV-infected women are no less likely to become pregnant than uninfected women (Ahluwalia, DeVellis, & Thomas, 1998; Pivnick, Jacobson, Eric, Mulvihill, Hsu, & Drucker, 1991;

(continued)

TABLE 4.1 Use of Reading Guide to Conduct an Initial Appraisal of a Research Report *(Continued)*

Literature review *(cont'd)*	Sunderland, Minkoff, Handte, Moroso, & Landesman, 1992). Further, although some have contended that HIV-infected women are more likely to choose to terminate their pregnancies than uninfected women (Jemmott & Miller, 1996), studies have consistently failed to find a significant difference in the tendency to have an abortion (Johnstone, Brettle, MacCallum, Mok, Peutherer, & Burns, 1990; Pivnick et al., 1991; Selwyn, Carter, Schoenbaum, Robertson, Klein, & Rogers, 1989; Sunderland et al., 1992). These studies, although representing a much needed first step in understanding the phenomenon of pregnancy among HIV-infected women, provided little insight into the reasons HIV-infected women choose to become pregnant.

Reasons for Pregnancy

Women's pregnancy desires and decisions may be influenced by a large number of psychological, social, and economic factors. Although most of the literature on pregnancy has focused on teen pregnancy or women with fertility problems, some work has examined the pregnancy desires of healthy adult women. One is Gerson's (1985) interviews with 63 primarily White women about their reasons for wanting a child. She demonstrated that both social and personal pressures influenced women's pregnancy decisions. Social pressures for having a child included men (husband/boyfriend) encouraging and pressuring the women and perceived social disapproval of childlessness. More personal reasons included women's fears that not having a child would lead to a lonely and desolate old age and the belief that not having a child would mean a loss of an important life experience. It is currently unknown whether the reasons these healthy (i.e., HIV-negative) women offered for wanting a child differ from those of women living with HIV/AIDS.

Few studies have investigated the factors that influence reproductive decisions of HIV-infected women. What research has examined this issue has tended to focus on the structural or demographic correlates or predictors of pregnancy. For example, Kline, Strickler, and Kempf (1995) found that among the 238 seropositive women they studied, multivariate analysis demonstrated that pregnancy was associated with younger age, more years since diagnosis, greater number of children, greater number of miscarriages, having a partner who wanted children, and having a partner with an

TABLE 4.1 *(Continued)*

unknown HIV status. Similarly, in a sample of 403 HIV-infected women studied, Bedimo, Bessinger, and Kissinger (1998) found that only a younger age and a history of sexual assault were significant predictors of pregnancy in multivariate analysis. Although demographic factors such as age, parental history, and disease characteristics, identified as predictors or correlates of pregnancy among HIV-infected women, may provide useful information regarding where to target educational campaigns, they do not offer insights into the reasons that underlie HIV-infected women's desire to have a baby. Furthermore, because demographic factors are not amenable to change, they do not offer the opportunities for intervention that knowledge of reasons for pregnancy may provide (e.g., by identifying and rectifying misinformation that may be the basis for decision making).

To date, there has been little research into the reasons infected women may desire a child, although some theoretical and descriptive work has begun (Armistead & Forehand, 1995; Jemmott & Miller, 1996; Murphy, Mann, O'Keefe, & Rotheram-Borus, 1998). To date, only two empirical studies have specifically addressed this question. In interviews with 49 HIV-positive women in New York City, Pivnick (1994) identified three major influences on pregnancy. These motives for having children included the desire to have something "of one's own" and the important cultural meaning children had for these women. A third reason was noted among women who already had children but had been separated from them for some period of time (e.g., lost custody due to drugs, homelessness, etc.). These women, who were more likely to desire to become pregnant than women who had not been separated from their children, felt that these children were not fully theirs or believed they could do a better job raising a child now.

Another focus group–based study of 22 HIV-infected women (Sowell & Misener, 1997), half of whom had been pregnant following their HIV diagnosis, identified several different factors that influenced pregnancy decisions or current desire to have a child. Among those factors supporting the desire for pregnancy were the women's faith that God would protect the child, past pregnancy experiences (e.g., previously having a healthy uninfected child), and feeling that a baby would make their lives complete. Factors discouraging pregnancy included a lack of awareness that the risk of

(continued)

TABLE 4.1 Use of Reading Guide to Conduct an Initial Appraisal of a
Research Report *(Continued)*

Literature review *(cont'd)*	perinatal transmission could be substantially reduced and concerns about the impact of pregnancy on their own health. The study also suggested that the feelings of family members and sexual partners, including the prospective father, had little impact on women's pregnancy decisions (Sowell & Misener, 1997). Although these two studies yielded important insights, the lack of correspondence in the findings suggests the need for additional studies to help clarify the reasons women living with HIV/AIDS may desire to become pregnant. *Many might view HIV-infected women as selfish or deviant for desiring a child or becoming pregnant. Because of this, it is especially important to give voice to these women's own reasons and justifications for their pregnancy. Further, an understanding of the reasons they offer for wanting pregnancy are crucial to gaining insight into the reproductive desires and decisions of HIV-infected women.*
Orientation toward target phenomenon	Justifications (Scott & Lyman, 1968) are reasons offered by an individual for why they believe their behavior is acceptable, although the behavior might be viewed as inappropriate or improper by others. These justifications provide insight into these women's own rationale and reasons for desiring a child.
Orientation toward inquiry	Many aspects of the design and analysis are consistent with a feminist perspective (e.g., Fine, 1992; Ussher, 1999). For example, central to the present research was the investigators' commitment to illuminating the women's lived experience by giving that experience expression in their own voices. The research also reflected an appreciation of the value and importance of understanding women's lay belief systems in trying to interpret meaningfully and explain their behavior. Finally, the research sought to illustrate the complexity of women's experiences by both illuminating the multiple determinants that shape their behavior and the diverse social contexts in which their actions are embedded.
Sampling strategy & techniques	To examine the reasons women offered for becoming pregnant or considering doing so in the future despite living with a life-threatening illness, interviews were conducted with a multiethnic sample of 51 HIV-infected women living in New York City. Potential participants were screened over the telephone to determine their eligibility. Women were eligible for inclusion in the study if they: (1) were between 20 and 45 years of age; (2) had tested seropositive for HIV antibodies; (3)

TABLE 4.1 *(Continued)*

	resided in the New York City metropolitan area; and 4) if Latina, were Puerto Rican (of any race) and had resided on the mainland for at least four years, or if African American or White, were native born and non-Hispanic; and 5) either were currently pregnant, attempting to become pregnant, or report that they were still open to the possibility of attempting pregnancy sometime in the future. The restriction to only Hispanic women of Puerto Rican decent was made because Puerto Rican women represent the majority of HIV-infected Latinas in New York City, and because inclusion of Latinas of other cultural backgrounds (e.g. Dominicans, Cubans) would introduce significant cultural variability such that meaningful comparisons could not be made. No restrictions were placed on past drug use or disease stage.
	Efforts were made to recruit Puerto Rican, African American, and White women from similar sources to avoid selection bias.
Sample size & composition	This resulted in a sample of 51 women living with HIV/AIDS. Sixty-five percent were African American, 23% were Puerto Rican, and 12% were non-Hispanic White. The mean age of the sample was 32.5 years ($SD = 5.1$). Forty-three percent of the women had less than a high school education, 18% had graduated high school, 26% had completed some college or professional training, and only 16% had completed an associate's degree or more. Sixty-three percent reported a household income of less than $15,000 per year. Thirty-one percent were married; 27% were divorced, separated, or widowed; and 41% reported they had never been married. However, many of the unmarried women (71%) lived with a partner or boyfriend. The women represented a number of religious affiliations, including Baptist (29%), Catholic (28%), and other Protestant denominations (14%). Nearly a quarter of the women (22%) reported an "other" religious affiliation (many of whom were Pentecostal), and only three women (6%) reported no religious affiliation. At the time of the interview, 29% of the women were HIV-asymptomatic, 26% were HIV-symptomatic, and 45% had been diagnosed with AIDS. Twenty-eight percent of the women reported past intravenous drug use.
	Most of the women were already mothers (67%) with between one and six children ($M = 2.38$, $SD = 1.41$). Of these, 62% had one or more children currently

(continued)

TABLE 4.1 Use of Reading Guide to Conduct an Initial Appraisal of a Research Report (*Continued*)

Sample size & composition *(cont'd)*	living with them. Eleven (22%) women were currently pregnant, 9 (18%) were trying to conceive, 6 (12%) were planning to attempt to conceive within the next year, and 25 (49%) were open to the possibility of a future pregnancy. Fifty-one percent of the women (including those currently pregnant) reported having been pregnant since their HIV diagnosis.
	Women were recruited from a diverse group of community settings, including HIV testing sites, women's health clinics, and HIV service organizations within the New York City metropolitan area.
Data collection or generation techniques & sources	Eligible women wishing to participate were scheduled for an interview at the investigators' research offices. *After obtaining informed consent, each woman participated in a focused interview* lasting approximately two hours. Interviews were conducted between January 1996 and April 1997, with the majority completed in early 1996—prior to the widespread use of protease inhibitor medications that have greatly improved the health of many HIV-infected individuals. The interviewers were female, Master's-level clinicians experienced in interviewing medically ill individuals.
	Focused interviews, as conceptualized by Merton, Fiske, and Kendall (1956), were conducted with all study participants. Consistent with this method, interviewers employed an interview guide or outline of topic areas developed by the researchers. The guide was not used as a formal interview schedule, but rather as a conceptual road map that provided points of reference throughout the interview. Interviewers were trained to follow the participants' lead and, when possible, use their comments as a bridge from one topic area to another. The interview guide contained questions about a broad range of topics relevant to women living with HIV/AIDS, including perceived risks and benefits of pregnancy, beliefs about transmission, and attitudes toward AZT during pregnancy. As the data gathering proceeded, the guide was modified to incorporate new insights gained into the phenomenon under investigation. The present analysis focuses on the women's responses to the question, "Can you tell me why you might want to become pregnant despite being HIV positive?"
Data management & analysis techniques	Interviews were audiotaped and transcribed for analysis. Transcripts ranged from 60 to 120 single-spaced pages. The data were then analyzed through a process of thematic content analysis (Krippendorff, 1981). The transcripts were read by the authors to identify themes

TABLE 4.1 *(Continued)*

reflecting the reasons women reported for becoming or wanting to become pregnant. Detailed notes were taken for each participant noting what reasons that individual offered for wanting to become pregnant and other contextual variables that may have influenced her pregnancy desire (e.g., number of children, partner status). The text was analyzed to examine if the women themselves reported being influenced by their ethnicity, current pregnancy status, or motherhood status. *The researchers developed a set of initial codes after each read a random sample of 20 interviews.*

Comparisons were made to examine if the types of reasons or justifications for pregnancy varied by ethnic/racial group, pregnancy status (i.e., currently pregnant or not), and motherhood status (i.e., already have children or not). Finally, quotations were selected by the researchers that they felt best represented the reasons offered by the sample for wanting/becoming pregnant. Direct quotations are presented below, when possible, to better represent the women's own voices.

The qualitative methods and analysis strategy employed in this study were not designed to derive reliable estimates of the true prevalence of the various reasons and beliefs identified as important to pregnancy desires. Because of the nature of the interviews, the content and time devoted to each topic varied considerably from participant to participant, depending on the woman's own salient concerns. Therefore, as in past work employing the same methodology, prevalence statistics have not been calculated. Rather, the goal of the present study was to generate insights, for which qualitative methods are well suited. Each theme reported, however, was found in at least 10 interviewees.

Orientation to & techniques for maximizing validity

Each interviewer participated in approximately 12 hours of training on nondirective interviewing, techniques to inquire or probe for more complete responses, and HIV-specific background information needed for the study (e.g., effectiveness of AZT to prevent perinatal transmission). In addition, interviewers each completed mock interviews. To ensure quality control throughout the data collection period, random interviews conducted by each interviewer were selected, reviewed, and feedback provided.

The researchers developed a set of initial codes after each read a random sample of 20 interviews. There was a very high agreement between the two researchers' initial codes (88% agreement) with seven of the eight

(continued)

TABLE 4.1 Use of Reading Guide to Conduct an Initial Appraisal of a Research Report *(Continued)*

Orientation to & techniques for maximizing validity *(cont'd)*	themes identified by both researchers. Consensus was reached between the two researchers on the final construction of these preliminary codes. The remaining interviews were then coded to determine if the coding scheme developed on the subsample was consistent with the remaining data, and if any additional reasons not identified in earlier interviews were present. No new themes were identified in the full sample of interviews. Inter-rater reliability for the coding was not computed because it was not believed to be meaningful for interviews of this nature (see Morse, 1997).
	A number of potential limitations of the present study must be acknowledged. Given that women had to self-refer into the study, it is possible that the study participants were more open about their HIV status than those who did not participate. Thus, the present sample may represent a selected sample of the population of younger HIV-infected women who experience less shame or fewer feelings of stigmatization. Such women may feel less constrained than others about social attitudes toward infected women becoming pregnant. Further, although the women's reports offer insight into factors that may influence their decision to become pregnant, future longitudinal and quantitative research will be required to link these reasons and justifications to actual pregnancy outcomes. Because the sample was restricted to women who were currently pregnant, attempting to become pregnant, or open to the future possibility of becoming pregnant, the study does not shed light on the perceived barriers and deterrents to pregnancy that may counterbalance women's reasons for desiring to become pregnant and their justifications for such a choice. Finally, recent developments in antiviral medications, such as the widespread use of protease inhibitors, have taken place since data collection. The potential implications this may have for women's consideration of pregnancy are currently unknown and need further research.
Findings	The decision to attempt pregnancy was not one that was made easily or taken lightly by these women. They struggled to weigh their desire to have a (or another) child against the potential risks involved. All of the women were primarily concerned with the possibility of having an HIV-infected child, and they also expressed fears about their own, and possibly the prospective father's, precarious health and the implications this might have for the child's care in the future. Some also worried that the pregnancy might further compromise

TABLE 4.1 *(Continued)*

their health and accelerate the progression of their disease. Thus, their desire for becoming pregnant was not based on a lack of knowledge or a failure to appreciate the inherent risks. Rather, despite the risks, these women expressed considerable interest in or desire to have a child, and in some cases were already pregnant.

Reasons for Wanting a Baby

Women reported a number of reasons—both personal and social—for wanting to have a baby. The explanations they offered appear similar to those one might hear from healthy women in their reproductive years. When cases were sorted by ethnic/racial group, by currently or not currently pregnant, or by motherhood status, almost none of the reasons were found to be exclusive to one subgroup. The only exception was one reason relevant only to women who had had children previously (see "I missed out on raising my other children" below). The distribution of reasons were similar across groups, although the sample was too small and the distribution of cases across subgroups too skewed to permit a meaningful statistical test of subgroup differences.

My husband/partner really wants children. Many women reported that their desire for a child was strongly influenced by the wishes of a husband or partner. For these women, having a child was a natural goal to pursue within the context of a loving relationship. They did not want HIV/AIDS to deter them from pursuing this goal, especially if their partner desired that they have a child together. For example, when asked why she wanted to have a baby, one woman explained:

> Well, the man I'm with, [boyfriend's name], I love him really much, which is kinda weird for me because I never felt this way about somebody so quick and he's like every girl's dream. And um, he has no children, he wants to and it just seems right, you know, to make a baby together. It just seems right. I think between me and him if we made a baby, she would be very pretty. She would have his hair, and she would just be a doll baby, and that would be his mom's first grand[child] and that's like important too. I think he would be a good father, because he's really good with my two [other children].

(continued)

TABLE 4.1 Use of Reading Guide to Conduct an Initial Appraisal of a Research Report *(Continued)*

Findings *(cont'd)*	Other women wanted to provide a child (particularly a son) to a husband who did not yet have children. Frequently, having a child was viewed as a "gift" that a woman could give her husband or boyfriend. When asked why she wished to have a child, one woman replied:

> Because of my husband. Because he wants a son so bad. And I want to be able to give it to him, you know . . . my husband, because he wants a son, you know. I mean I want a baby for him. I do want to have my husband's baby, but I just don't want to have it right now. We just got married. We're going on three months. But I will give him one. But if I get pregnant, yes I'll have the baby, you know, it wouldn't make a difference. [What doesn't make a difference?] Being HIV. It doesn't have anything to do—it doesn't matter. It doesn't matter to him. Before I met him I wouldn't have had no more babies, you know. But since I met him, I want another baby. And being HIV doesn't matter to me, because it doesn't matter to him.

In some cases, it appeared that the husbands or boyfriends exerted a great deal of pressure on the woman to have a baby, causing tension within the relationship. This was because women felt that they would feel guilty and profoundly upset if they acceded to the partner's wishes and the child were to be infected. As one woman commented:

> There's a lot of things that goes through your head, both positive and negative. It's like, I started thinking about my husband saying he always wanted a baby, but I still would have that guilt in me. How my baby's gonna be born, how he's gonna feel when he raised. up? All these things. [Have you talked to your husband about those feelings?] Yeah, and he say "Well okay, let's stop trying." But I could see it on he face. He's disappointed. And that makes me feel guilty. Like he really wants it, and I feel like if I stop, it be all right with him, but in another way it would hurt him. And he got the hope high that he want a baby. So, I'm willing to have it, if it comes.

I missed out on raising my other children. Another reason, offered only by women who had previously had children, was that they wanted to have another baby because they felt that they had missed out on some important parts of their child's life because of separations associated with their histories of drug use,

TABLE 4.1 *(Continued)*

homelessness, and prostitution. Typically, during these separations, children had been placed in foster care or with a relative who had assumed legal custody. Some of the women had never regained custody of their children, leaving them feeling childless and wanting a child of their own so that they could enjoy certain experiences of parenthood that they had never had with their other children. However, even those who had regained custody of their child(ren) felt they had missed something very important.

> Before I went into recovery my son was removed from my care from the age of six months till two years. And so I missed some very good months and um, yeah, I feel remorseful, because I would have liked to have been with him. After my diagnosis, I didn't think it would be fair to bring another child into this world. But then I thought about it, thinking that I would like to have a baby that I could nurture in the early years. So I thought about it, I'm considering it. It was like, when he was a baby I didn't have him but two weeks [before he was put in foster care]. So it wasn't like no time at all. So I missed out with him and his brother. All of my kids were taken from me at one point during my drug use. That was my fault, and I understand that now, but I missed out having little babies.

The importance of these lost moments and experiences was so profound that some women felt that their child(ren) were not fully theirs because they had not raised them continuously.

> I'm a more responsible person now. I didn't take care of my other four children you know, raising them. I had them for a while when they were maybe up until about five or six years old, and you know that was a really beautiful part of my life and their life. And I would just, you know, I just would like to have a baby that I can like really call mine. Because in some way I don't really call them mine because I didn't really raise them.

A child will enable me to feel complete, fulfilled, and happy. Another reason often cited by the women for wanting to have a child was the belief that it would make them feel complete, fulfilled, and very happy. For those who had already had children, taking care of a newborn was remembered as one of the happiest times in their lives—a happiness they wished to relive. For example,

(continued)

TABLE 4.1 Use of Reading Guide to Conduct an Initial Appraisal of a Research Report *(Continued)*

Findings *(cont'd)*	It's just having a baby it makes me so happy. Taking care of a baby and just the whole process of the whole thing. It makes me so happy. That's like the most happiest times throughout my whole life has been having children. The closeness, just knowing that I'm needed and they depend on me, it's something that makes me feel great. That makes me happy, that they need me. That I have to be there and I have to take care of them and they need to be fed. It fulfills me, my mind, mentally, spiritually, and within my gut, my soul, I feel full. You know it makes me feel that I wasn't just put on this world to be here, I was here for a reason.

For those women who had not yet had a child, having a baby was part of a cherished life dream they greatly wished to fulfill. Many held a romanticized view of family life, which they felt that having a child would help them realize. For example,

> I don't know, it's like you just have this thing in your mind as a child. You want to grow up and get married, go to college, get a house and a car and a dog, and you know, children. It just makes your life complete.

> I love kids. I didn't just want one kid. Babies just make you happy. They do. I love babies. I'll babysit anybody's baby for them. Don't even pay me, just let me play with the kid. That's the number one reason.

Others felt that if they could have a child, their lives would feel more complete. Although the women did not speak in terms of the social pressures or the cultural importance of children, some did express that they viewed having children as a natural and important part of being a woman.

> I know life would be more complete. I feel like I would be finally complete. There's a missing piece to this puzzle. I have a husband. I have a beautiful apartment. I am starting school next week. I'm going to start counseling, you know, training to be a counselor. My husband's going back to work. I have my cat, a wonderful family. I'd be so complete with a baby in the picture. A child to send to school and just love and nurture.

> Well, felt that I would be a complete woman. I would never have experienced a full meaning of

TABLE 4.1 *(Continued)*

womanhood without having a child. Giving birth to a child and nurturing a child. And giving a child my values and teaching it what I know. Leaving something to the world that's hopefully something positive.

Justifications for Wanting a Baby

In addition to their reasons for wanting a child, the women spontaneously expressed a number of beliefs that they felt helped to justify their desire for a baby despite having a life-threatening illness that could be transmitted to the child. Justifications, as originally defined by Scott and Lyman (1968), are reasons offered by an individual for why they believe their behavior is acceptable, although the behavior might be viewed as inappropriate or stigmatized by others. Although we did ask the women what their reasons for wanting to become pregnant were, we did not specifically ask them to justify their desires. Rather, they spontaneously offered these comments in the form of justifications. These justifications appeared to serve a very important role in women's willingness to consider becoming pregnant or having become pregnant. Often these women appeared to be justifying their desire for pregnancy to themselves as well as our interviewers. Women frequently offered multiple justifications. No differences in the justifications offered were noted among the three ethnic/racial groups or between women who were currently or not currently pregnant or those who already had children and those who did not. Nearly all of the justifications appeared to address the women's concern about having an HIV-infected child by offering reasons why they believed they could have a healthy baby. Other justifications reflected the women's view that the current prospects for an infected woman having a healthy baby were considerably improved over the past.

Other infected women have had healthy babies. Many of these women reported being personally acquainted with or having heard about other HIV-infected women who had given birth to a healthy baby or whose baby had seroconverted (i.e., was born with HIV antibodies, but never had the virus and now was HIV-negative). This knowledge was very empowering for the women and helped to support their belief that it was possible for infected women, like themselves, to have healthy babies.

(continued)

TABLE 4.1 Use of Reading Guide to Conduct an Initial Appraisal of a Research Report *(Continued)*

Findings *(cont'd)*	Sometimes I think I can't do it, but then I got to have some faith and have some positive attitude that it can be done. Because I know somebody that's HIV-positive. She had a baby. The baby came out big, fat and healthy, but it was HIV positive. Two months later they took the test again for the baby and it is not positive. Now that baby is bigger and prettier than ever. The baby's fine. I think that could happen to me.
	The two [HIV-positive] women I know, their children, the one is two and the other is three. Their children are negative. They were positive, but they're negative now. . . . And well, that's made me feel even a little better to know somebody personally, as opposed to reading about it or seeing a documentary or something.
	The lady who told me her baby was okay, that influenced me. She told me, "You gonna be okay," and um, she just mentioned, "I have a baby," and she showed me a picture and she said "My baby's okay." [And why was that so important?] That gave me the inspiration to know that it can happen, that if you do take that chance and get pregnant, that the baby will be okay. It gave me that incentive. I look at it that way. I have a great chance of him not being positive.
	The opinions and experiences of other HIV-positive women carried a great deal of weight. In contrast to physicians or family (who they often suggested had not influenced their desires), other infected women were viewed as peers whose experiences and opinions were more trusted and seen as personally relevant. For example, in response to a query about who had been most influential in her thinking about having a baby, one woman said:
	It's just basically like two girlfriends of me that knows that I was thinking—that I talked to them about it. These girls that I go to my clinic with and they pregnant too. They influenced me to keep it. [Why have their opinions been so important to you?] Because there is no better opinion to take than someone who's actually going through the experience. And they've lived through it. You know, so their opinion means a lot because they're actually going through it and one of them already had one that had HIV converted [became

TABLE 4.1 *(Continued)*

> HIV-negative], and she's very optimistic about the second one. So, I think everything is going to be okay for me too.

Not only were women influenced by knowing other HIV-infected women who had healthy children, but those who had themselves given birth to healthy babies since being infected frequently advocated to other HIV-infected women that they too could have a healthy baby. For example,

> I know a lot of women out there who are HIV-positive and they want to have a child. And these women, they cry with me in the group how they can't because they'll have an infected baby. You know, and I give them my opinion. Look at me. I did it. You know, there's some place for everything you do in this life. And to me, faith had a lot to do with it. So I suggest they do the same because the decision is up to them. Being positive or not being positive, if you want a child, it makes no sense not to. There are so many things going on now, the medications work. It worked for me. And the decision was solely mine. The same way the decision should be solely theirs.

<u>AZT can help me have a healthy baby.</u> At the time, the recent finding that the risk of vertical transmission (i.e., infection from mother to child) could be substantially reduced through a regimen of maternal and infant use of the antiviral medication AZT was viewed by the women as removing or at least diminishing a significant earlier deterrent to pregnancy. Numerous women expressed that they would never want to have a child suffer with this disease. They felt, however, that because there was now a highly effective, though not perfect, preventive treatment available, the risk of having an infected child was acceptably small now, whereas previously it might not have been. Consequently, they felt it was no longer inappropriate to consider pregnancy.

> Before the information about AZT came out, I saw the risk as being 25% to 30%, and it was well absolutely not, that's way too big a risk. But when all of this information about AZT became available, both my husband and I talked about it and we were really excited about it and thought, humm, well, a 10% or 8% risk, maybe we can do that and just pray that we're not in that 10%, and sort of stay inclined to open up the potential of having a baby.

(continued)

TABLE 4.1 Use of Reading Guide to Conduct an Initial Appraisal of a Research Report *(Continued)*

Findings *(cont'd)*	
	Until they came out with the possibility of administering AZT while a woman is pregnant, I had already decided I was not going to have a child. I was considering attempting to adopt. I was preparing to have a tubal ligation. But they kept telling me here at the gyn clinic that I was too young, and why would I even consider it. But once I found out about the results—the possible results, I had changed my mind and I said okay. Now I'm willing to try. Once I heard about the results I said well now I can attempt to have my own child rather than adopt.
	<u>I have faith in God.</u> Several of the women who were religious used their faith not only in coping with the everyday stresses of the illness, but also in helping to direct their lives. Thus, it is not surprising that many offered their faith in God as a strong influence on their pregnancy decision making. These women often discounted the risks of vertical transmission, believing that God would protect the child from being HIV-infected.
	Now I want to have a child because I know, I have faith in God, you know what I'm saying; that I was blessed that my last baby didn't come out positive. I have it in my heart that I know I'm going to have a healthy baby, so I'm trying not to think negative. I want to think positive. But if it happens [the baby is infected], I'm still going to love it just the same.
	When the time comes for me to get pregnant, I believe that I will get pregnant. And I believe that the child will be born not infected. I mean that's just something—like I was saying about God. I mean, God is sovereign. He does what he wants to do. I know that even though I've done what I've done to get this [HIV], I believe that he will be just, and not let my child become HIV positive. I really do. And I just feel that so strongly that I'm just gonna leave it in fate and see what happens.
	Today I have faith that I am going to live. I know that God is going to bless me with a child. I know my child ain't going to suffer and he's going to have or he or she is going to have the good things I never had. He won't suffer with HIV, with this disease.
	Others entirely relinquished control over their pregnancy to God. These women believed that God would not

TABLE 4.1 *(Continued)*

allow them to become pregnant if it was wrong or if it would result in a sick child. To these women, babies were viewed as gifts from God, provided to women who were doing "the right thing":

> I didn't know what I should do. So I decided to take it to—to God in prayer. And I said "God, if it's your will, I will get pregnant. And if I don't, then I will accept that." And after about a month after I took this in prayer, I was pregnant after 15 years of nothing. So that made me think that I was, you know, doing the right thing.

> I'll leave it in God's hands. I mean, you know, if it wasn't meant for me to get pregnant, God wouldn't put it there. Evidently it was meant for me to be pregnant. I strongly believe in God, I believe that. And I know He's a healer and I believe He can heal me from this, if I do the right thing.

The belief that whether they would have a healthy child, or even become pregnant, was in God's hands, allowed some women to believe it was all right to forego using condoms to prevent pregnancy, or to take AZT to help prevent transmission to the baby if they became pregnant. Their belief that God's wishes would be served by whatever happened enabled women to relinquish control of any pregnancy decisions and shift responsibility for whether they became pregnant and the outcome of that pregnancy to God.

I am still healthy and young. Contrary to current medical views, some women felt that the chances of having a healthy child could be even further increased if they stayed in good health during pregnancy and took care of themselves. Many believed that if they were going to have a child, they should do it while they were still young and "healthy." That is, these women believed that as their disease progressed (T cells lowering, viral load increasing) the risks of transmission of the virus to the baby would increase. They also believed that older age in general was associated with more risks of having an unhealthy child.

> Something in the back of my mind keeps telling me you're 30 years old, your biological clock is ticking, and my T cell count is still high. I'm in the 1,100 range. So I don't want to wait until I get much older and my body gets weaker and then the chances of transmitting it to the baby would be greater, so I figure now is the time if I'm going to do it.

(continued)

TABLE 4.1 Use of Reading Guide to Conduct an Initial Appraisal of a Research Report *(Continued)*

Findings *(cont'd)*	My T cell count is so high, and I haven't experienced any of the opportunistic diseases. So I feel that the chance would be greater for me to have a healthy child, because I'm not so sickly and my body is healthy. So I figure my chances are much more greater to have a healthy child now.

There's like a time clock clicking in my head. Like I may be physically able to have this child now, but who's to say in six months from now, everything could turn around and I won't be able to carry the baby full term or have a healthy child. So that's another thing too. The clock is ticking, so if I'm going to do something, it's best that I do it now and go ahead with it.

I am better able to raise a child now. A number of women felt that because they had stopped using drugs (often in response to their HIV diagnosis) they were now, in some cases for the first time in their adult lives, responsible enough to care for a child. Ironically, although some had never considered motherhood before their diagnosis because of their lifestyle, they now felt it appropriate for them to contemplate that possibility. Often, those who wanted to have another child because of missing out on some part of their children's lives justified that desire by arguing that they felt that they were far better able to care for a child now than they had been earlier.

Because of my active addiction, I missed a lot of my three children growing up. But this would give me a chance to be able, because I'm clean now, to raise this one fully, without being under the influence of anything.

I want a baby so bad. I think that at this time in my life, I've stopped doing drugs, I've stopped doing alcohol. I've really turned my life around. I did a 360-degree with my life. I've educated myself and I help others today. I think that that's one of the things that I really want.

I made a lot of mistakes when I had my son before. I don't know, it would be like to make up or try to do it right this time maybe. Maybe in a sense it would be for that too. To try to get it right this time. Do things differently.

Others were in a stable relationship with a partner for the first time in many years. These changes led them to perceive their situation as one that would provide suitable circumstances for contemplating having a child.

TABLE 4.1 *(Continued)*

Well first of all, with my children, I was never married. If I were to get pregnant, this would be my first child that's not born out of wedlock. And I'm in a much healthier, happy relationship. This time I would have someone that would help me raise my children, because I raised the other three by myself.

I've gotten my life together. I have a great relationship with my boyfriend. I've always wanted to be a mother, but I was just too wrapped up in myself and hanging out and partying to ever consider it. I also like the fact of looking at a little me. Just the thought of having a child makes me smile. The joy of having someone that is mine, all mine, you know. This came from me. This is my baby, and just having those little things like "Mommie, I'm home" or kisses and those little "Mommie, I love you" and stuff like that. I've missed all these years, being so selfish, wrapped in myself. Now that life is all behind me, it's something that I really would like to enjoy before I leave this earth.

Logic & form of findings	Experimental style Thematic, ordered by reasons and justifications; use of in vivo phrases as headers
Discussion & implications	The present study provides additional insights into the psychosocial factors associated with HIV-infected women's desire to become pregnant despite their illness. Although the choice to attempt conception while living with HIV/AIDS has been viewed by others as short-sighted or selfish, these desires and decisions need to be understood from the perspective of the women making this choice.
	These women recognized that the decision to bear a child while infected carried risks for the child, as well as for themselves and their partners. However, they also felt a strong desire for a child.
	Some of the reasons the women offered for desiring a child were similar to those that might be found among their healthier peers in their reproductive years, such as the wanting to satisfy the wishes of husbands or partners or the belief that a child would bring a sense of fulfillment and completeness (Gerson, 1985). A number of the reasons identified among these HIV-infected women were also quite similar to those reported in an earlier study of women's feelings about pregnancy following breast cancer treatment (Siegel, Gorey, & Gluhoski, 1997). Women with breast cancer also

(continued)

TABLE 4.1 Use of Reading Guide to Conduct an Initial Appraisal of a
Research Report *(Continued)*

Discussion & Implications *(cont'd)*	reported both that their desire for a child was influenced by their husband's wishes and that having a child was part of a cherished life dream they wished to realize and that would fulfill them in a unique way. This suggests that women, regardless of their health or illness, may hold similar reasons for wanting a child.

The present findings are also consistent with prior work on pregnancy among HIV-infected women. Consistent with Pivnick (1994), we found that women who had been separated from their children, even temporarily, wanted another chance to raise a child so that they could fully experience the joys of motherhood and parent this new child better than they had their previous children. Like Sowell and Misener (1997), we found that some HIV-infected women reported that they were placing their faith in God to protect any child they might have against becoming infected. They also found, as we did, that women felt that a child would fulfill them and make their lives more complete. However, while Sowell and Misener (1997) explicitly remarked that husbands and family had little influence on women's pregnancy decisions, our data confirmed Kline and colleagues' (1995) finding on the importance of a partner's wishes for a child. However, consistent with Sowell and Misener (1997), family (i.e., parents and siblings) and physicians were found to have little influence in the present study. Thus, the great similarity of the present findings to previous work lends greater confidence to the validity of these findings.

In addition to reporting their reasons for wanting to have a child, the women also frequently offered "justifications" (Scott & Lyman, 1968) or explanations for why they believed a pregnancy was an acceptable and responsible choice despite their illness. Although women were never asked to justify their desires, these reasons were spontaneously offered for why pregnancy was an acceptable choice. Perhaps, because these women were very aware of the public attitudes against HIV-infected women becoming pregnant, these women felt the need or had previously needed to defend their desires. However, it appeared that these women were using these justifications to justify their desires to "themselves" as well. These justifications also appeared to be very important in enabling the women to feel more comfortable with their desire to have a baby. Unlike the reasons for desiring a child, many of these justifications were specific to the HIV/AIDS context. The overarching theme of the majority of the justifications

TABLE 4.1 *(Continued)*

offered was to provide explanations for why the women believed they could now have a healthy baby (e.g., God would protect the baby, other women have had healthy babies, I am healthy so I am more likely to have a healthy baby, AZT can help me have a healthy baby).

One previously unreported justification offered for becoming pregnant or contemplating pregnancy stemmed from the recent finding that an antiviral medication regimen (AZT) reduced the risk of mother-to-child transmission of infection. Many women felt that this reduction in transmission rates was sufficiently low to make pregnancy an acceptable risk and was justification enough to consider pregnancy. It should be noted, however, that although the women viewed the finding that AZT could significantly reduce the risk of perinatal transmission as a very positive development, many continued to have negative attitudes about the side effects of AZT and the risks associated with its toxicity. Others were concerned about the danger exposure to AZT posed for the baby or were uncertain if it would benefit the child. Indeed, a number of women felt that the 25% risk of transmission found among women not using the AZT regimen was sufficiently favorable odds for them to risk pregnancy without taking the antiviral regimen.

Consistent with earlier work on health behaviors and health decision-making, the present study suggests that the experiences and beliefs of other HIV-infected women may be very important in choosing to become pregnant. Previous work has suggested that peer beliefs and experiences may more strongly influence health behaviors and attitudes—such as those associated with medication adherence—than professional advice or recommendations (Siegel & Gorey, 1997; Siegel, Schrimshaw, & Raveis, 2000). The finding that discussions with other HIV-infected women who have had a healthy child were very important to other women's pregnancy desires suggests that beliefs about pregnancy (and its risks and benefits) are socially transmitted. Further evidence for the influence of interpersonal factors on attitudes toward childbearing exists in the women's reports of wishing to please their husbands/partners as one reason for desiring to become pregnant. Future research should explore more systematically the role of other possible interpersonal sources of influence on pregnancy decision-making, such as family, peers, and one's health care providers.

(continued)

TABLE 4.1 Use of Reading Guide to Conduct an Initial Appraisal of a Research Report *(Continued)*

Discussion & Implications *(cont'd)*	Of particular interest is the function that religious faith played in these women's reproductive decisions. Weighing the desire for a child against the risks of pregnancy left many women with great uncertainty as to what reproductive decision to make. For some, the responsibility for their desires and actions was reduced or eliminated by relinquishing to God control over both whether they become pregnant and the consequences for the child's health. By placing faith in God to protect the unborn child and to only allow pregnancy to occur if God felt it was the right thing to happen, the women reduced their conflict about becoming pregnant. This belief in the protective power of faith in some cases also diminished the motivation to use contraception, as well as the perceived need to take AZT to prevent transmission of the virus to the unborn child. Although religious faith was found to greatly influence many women on their contraception and pregnancy desires, its significance within other more religiously diverse samples must be explored. The heavily Baptist, Pentecostal, and Catholic sample obtained here may exhibit a greater faith in the healing and protective power of God than women affiliated with other religious denominations. Clearly the role of religiosity and/or religious denomination on pregnancy decisions as well as other health behaviors merits further exploration.
	Perhaps as notable as the reasons and justifications offered for considering becoming pregnant were those that were not offered. For example, it was expected that like breast cancer survivors (Siegel et al., 1997), HIV-infected women would report wanting a child because they wanted to feel "normal" and be involved in the same developmental tasks (child-rearing) as their peers. Although a couple of women suggested this as part of their motivation for wanting a baby, it was not a frequent or salient theme among the study sample. Another reason that was anticipated but not identified within the interviews was wanting a child in order to have someone who offered them unconditional love and who depended on them. Finally, in contrast to expectations, we found no differences in the nature of the reasons and justifications offered by currently pregnant women and those who felt they might desire to become pregnant in the future. Nor were any ethnic/racial differences observed or differences with respect to whether or not the women already had had any children (with the above noted exception).

TABLE 4.1 *(Continued)*

However, due to the small sample of White women and of currently pregnant women, the assertion that no differences exist cannot be made with certainty.

Implications

The findings have a number of implications for supportive interventions with HIV-infected women. In cases where the husband or partner's desire for a child is the principal motive, women should be helped to explore the stability of the relationship and the likely availability of the prospective father to help in the care and raising of the child. Women should also be encouraged to explore the strength of their own desire for a child independent of the partner and how they would feel if they had a child to please the partner and he subsequently left the relationship. Further, previous research suggested that many HIV-infected women feel that because of their illness they have very restricted opportunities for a relationship with a man. Thus, they are often willing to "settle" for a relationship that is unsatisfying in a number of ways. Women need to be encouraged to examine if they are considering having a baby to please their partner out of a fear of losing him if they do not accede to his wishes. Their emotional and sometimes financial dependence on their partner could obviously make them fearful of denying the partner's wishes even when they may not share the strong desire for a child.

With effective treatments, a supportive social network, and adequate information regarding the potential risks of pregnancy, HIV-infected women can make informed decisions regarding pregnancy, take preventative steps to reduce possible transmission to the child, and likely give birth to a healthy baby. Indeed, with current treatments available, this is probable. However, to make informed decisions women must be aware not only of the risks associated with pregnancy, but also must have inaccurate information or beliefs dispelled. The justifications offered by these women suggest a number of misconceptions, which may need to be directly challenged in future educational efforts. For example, the belief that being young or "healthy" will help reduce the risk of HIV transmission is unfounded. However, through promotion of accurate knowledge about risks and benefits of pregnancy, women living with HIV/AIDS may be empowered to make confident and fully informed decisions regarding pregnancy.

(continued)

TABLE 4.1 Use of Reading Guide to Conduct an Initial Appraisal of a Research Report *(Continued)*

Protection of human subjects	Participants were recruited through advertisements, flyers, and referrals from these organizations. In order to preserve confidentiality, women interested in participating in the research or wanting further information about the study were directed to telephone the research office.
	After obtaining informed consent, each woman participated in a focused interview.
	Women were told that we were interested in their thoughts about being/becoming pregnant while HIV-infected, about their knowledge of the risks, if any, having a baby might pose to themselves or the baby, as well as what they believed were the possible risks and benefits of taking AZT during pregnancy.
	Women were asked if they preferred an interviewer of their same race/ethnicity, and ethnically matched interviewers were provided for all women who expressed such a preference. Puerto Rican participants were interviewed by a bilingual interviewer. Each participant was reimbursed $25 for the research meeting and travel expenses.
Reviewer's abstract & summary appraisal	**Research purpose:** To describe HIV-positive women's reasons and justifications for having children
	Theoretical framework: Scott & Lyman justifications
	Method: Generic, descriptive
	Sample size & key characteristics: 51 (33 African American, 12 Puerto Rican, 6 White); primarily minority
	Data collection techniques: Interview
	Data analysis techniques: Content analysis
	Primary topic of findings: Reasons and justifications for having a child
	Secondary topics of findings: None
	Type of findings: Thematic survey
	Edited findings:
	Reasons for wanting a baby
	1. My husband/partner really wants children.
	2. I missed out on raising my other children.
	3. A child will enable me to feel complete, fulfilled, and happy.
	The decision to attempt pregnancy was not made easily or taken lightly.
	Women struggled to weigh their desire to have a (or another) child against the potential risks involved.
	All women were primarily concerned with the possibility of having an HIV-infected child.

TABLE 4.1 *(Continued)*

Women expressed fears about their own, and possibly the prospective father's, precarious health and the implications this might have for the child's care in the future.

Some women worried that the pregnancy might further compromise their health and accelerate the progression of their disease.

Women's desire for becoming pregnant was not based on a lack of knowledge or a failure to appreciate the inherent risks.

Despite the risks, women expressed considerable interest in or desire to have a child, and in some cases were already pregnant.

HIV-positive women's reasons for wanting a baby were similar to healthy women's reasons.

Reasons for having a child did not vary with parity or ethnicity.

Justifications for wanting a baby
1. Other infected women have had healthy babies.
2. AZT can help me have a healthy baby.
3. I have faith in God.
4. I am still healthy and young
5. I am better able to raise a child now.

In addition to reasons, women spontaneously offered justifications for wanting a child despite having a life-threatening illness that could be transmitted to the child.

These justifications appeared to serve a very important role in women's willingness to consider becoming pregnant or having become pregnant.

Often these women appeared to be justifying their desire for pregnancy to themselves as well as to us.

Women frequently offered multiple justifications.

No differences in justifications offered were noted by ethnicity or parity.

Justifications appeared to address the women's concern about having an HIV-infected child by offering reasons why they believed they could have a healthy baby.

Other justifications reflected the women's view that the current prospects for an HIV-positive woman having a healthy baby were considerably improved over the past.

The belief that whether they would have a healthy child, or even become pregnant, was in God's hands allowed some women to believe it was all right to forego using condoms to prevent pregnancy, or to take AZT to help prevent transmission to the baby if they became pregnant.

(continued)

TABLE 4.1 Use of Reading Guide to Conduct an Initial Appraisal of a Research Report *(Continued)*

Reviewer's abstract & summary appraisal *(cont'd)*	Another justification (especially among drug users) was the belief that they were better able to raise a child now.
	Evaluation: Acceptable
	Summary comments: Well-detailed and supported description with light infusions of theory and method.

Note. Repeated information is italicized. The reference list appearing at the end of this article is not included here. Minor revisions of style, and corrections of minor errors in spelling or wording appearing in the original report, have been made.

TABLE 4.2 Illustration of a Cross-Study Display for Comparative Appraisal

Report	Affiliation	Theory	Method	Type of findings	Form	Sampling plan	Sample
Barnes et al., 1997	Social work	Feminist, marginalized groups	Grounded theory	Interpretive explanation	Largely experimental	Convenience	12 (7AA, 4W, 1H)
Chin & Kroesen, 1999	Psychiatry & biobehavioral science	None specified; lean to gender & culture	Multimethod/ Grounded theory for analysis	Thematic	Experimental	Subsample from larger quantitative study	9 (all A/PI)
Ciambrone, 1999	Sociology	Biographical disruption	Feminism	Thematic	Amended experimental	Convenience	37 (23 W, 11 AA, 3H) See Ciambrone, 2001, 2002
Ciambrone, 2001	Sociology	Biographical disruption	None explicitly stated; Grounded theory references	Thematic	Amended experimental	Convenience	37 (23 W, 11 AA, 3H) See Ciambrone, 1999, 2002
Ciambrone, 2002	Sociology	Biographical disruption	Qualitative; Grounded theory references	Thematic	Amended experimental	Not stated	37 (23 W, 11 AA, 3H) See Ciambrone, 1999, 2001
Grove et al., 1997	Sociology	Bourdieu social capital	Ethnographic (in abstract); no method citations	Interpretive explanation	Amended experimental	Not stated	22 (18 W + 4 unspecified minority)

(continued)

TABLE 4.2 Illustration of a Cross-Study Display for Comparative Appraisal (*Continued*)

Report	Affiliation	Theory	Method	Type of findings	Form	Sampling plan	Sample
Ingram, 1996	Nursing	Opotow moral exclusion theory	Grounded theory	Interpretive explanation	Experimental	Theoretical	20 (11 W, 8 AA, 1 H) See Ingram & Hutchinson, 1999a, b, 2000
Ingram & Hutchinson, 1999a	Nursing	Cultural norm of motherhood	Grounded theory	Conceptual description	Largely experimental	Purposive	18 (9 W, 8 AA, 1 H) See Ingram, 1996, Ingram & Hutchinson, 1999b, 2000
Ingram & Hutchinson, 1999b	Nursing	Goffman stigma	Grounded theory	Thematic	Largely experimental	Volunteer	18 (9 W, 8 AA, 1 H) See Ingram, 1996, Ingram & Hutchinson, 1999a, 2000
Ingram & Hutchinson, 2000	Nursing	Bateson double bind	Grounded theory	Conceptual description	Largely experimental	Purposive	20 (11 W, 8 AA, 1 H) See Ingram, 1996, Ingram & Hutchinson, 1999b, 2000

Note. Shading is to show related samples. Complete citations are in the Appendix. AA=African American; W=White; H=Hispanic; A/PI=Asian/Pacific Islander.

REFERENCES

Atkinson, P., & Delamont, S. (2005). Analytic perspectives. In N. K. Denzin & Y. S. Lincoln (Eds.), *The Sage handbook of qualitative research* (3rd ed., pp. 821–840). Thousand Oaks, CA: Sage.

Barroso, J., & Sandelowski, M. (2003). Sample reporting in qualitative studies of women with HIV infection. *Field Methods, 15,* 386–404.

Bazerman, C. (1988). *Shaping written knowledge: The genre and activity of the experimental article in science.* Madison: University of Wisconsin Press.

Eakin, J. M., & Mykhalovskiy, E. (2003). Reframing the evaluation of qualitative health research: Reflections on a review of appraisal guidelines on the health sciences. *Journal of Evaluation in Clinical Practice, 9,* 187–194.

Edwards, A., Elwyn, G., Hood, K., & Rollnick, S. (2000). Judging the "weight of evidence" in systematic reviews: Introducing rigor into the qualitative overview stage by assessing signal and noise. *Journal of Evaluation in Clinical Practice, 6,* 177–184.

Edwards, A. G., Russell, I. T., & Stott, N. C. (1998). Signal versus noise in the evidence base for medicine: An alternative to hierarchies of evidence? *Family Practice, 15,* 319–322.

Golden-Biddle, K., & Locke, K. (1993). Appealing work: An investigation of how ethnographic texts convince. *Organization Science, 4,* 595–616.

Greenhalgh, T., Robert, G., Macfarlane, F., Bate, P., Kyriakidou, O., & Peacock, R. (2005). Storylines of research in diffusion of innovation: A meta-narrative approach to systematic review. *Social Science & Medicine, 61,* 417–430.

Gusfield, J. (1976). The literary rhetoric of science: Comedy and pathos in drinking driver research. *American Sociological Review, 41,* 16–34.

Johnson, M., Long, T., & White, A. (2001). Arguments for "British Pluralism" in qualitative health research. *Journal of Advanced Nursing, 33,* 243–249.

Manguel, A. (1996). *A history of reading.* Toronto: Knopf.

Richardson, L. (2000). Writing: A method of inquiry. In N. K. Denzin & Y. S. Lincoln (Eds.), *Handbook of qualitative research* (2nd ed., pp. 923–948). Thousand Oaks, CA: Sage.

Sandelowski, M. (2004). Using qualitative research. *Qualitative Health Research, 14,* 1366–1386.

Sandelowski, M., & Barroso, J. (2002). Reading qualitative studies. *International Journal of Qualitative Methods, 1(1),* Article 5. Retrieved December 15, 2002, from www.ualberta.ca/~ijqm/english/engframeset.html

Thorne, S., Joachim, G., Paterson, B., & Canam, C. (2002). Influence of the research frame on qualitatively derived health science knowledge. *International Journal of Qualitative Methods, 1(1),* Article 1. Retrieved December 15, 2002, from www.ualberta.ca/~ijqm/english/engframeset.html

Thorne, S., Paterson, B., Acorn, S., Canam, C., Joachim, G., & Jillings, C. (2002). Chronic illness experience: Insights from a metastudy. *Qualitative Health Research, 12,* 437–452.

CHAPTER FIVE

Classifying the Findings in Qualitative Research Reports

We have been emphasizing the reciprocal relationship between content and form in the research report. We turn now to the importance of understanding what researchers actually did in their studies ("logic-in-use"), as opposed to the claims they made in their reports of those studies ("reconstructed logic"; Kaplan, 1964, p. 8). Our intent is not to fault researchers, but rather to help reviewers address the problem that a perceived discrepancy between claims and actions poses for the appraisal process in qualitative research synthesis studies. The classification system, or typology, shown in Figure 5.1, will help you better understand the research findings in the reports you review. You will recall that findings constitute the primary data in qualitative research synthesis studies. The typology we present here will help you discern—in the research findings themselves—the actual methods used to produce them, and to select the techniques most suitable for integrating them. The use of this typology is a key component of the individual appraisal of reports we described in chapter 4. You can read more about the development of this typology in Sandelowski and Barroso (2003).

REWRITING THE TEXT

Because it is focused on the findings themselves, and not on researchers' claims about how they were produced, the typology allows for the inclusion in qualitative research synthesis projects of reports of studies containing findings that do not embody the stated method. For example, it

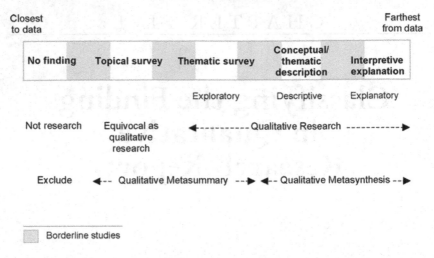

FIGURE 5.1 Types of qualitative research findings by integration method.

allows you to read what you consider to be misrepresented as the result of a hermeneutic analysis instead as the result of a content analysis. This is an example of the reader generosity we referred to in chapter 4 and of how readers may legitimately rewrite texts to preserve their utility. Undermining the validity of qualitative research synthesis studies is the exclusion of reports for reasons that do not adversely affect the credibility of the findings.

Indeed, leading scholars in the research synthesis field as a whole have warned against a "checklist mindset" toward quality (Barbour, 2001), and the exclusion (Conn & Rantz, 2003; Cooper, 1998) or "censorship" of reports because of "a priori prejudices" (Glass, 2000, p. 10). They have argued against a "best evidence" (Slavin, 1995) model for research synthesis whereby reviewers establish—a priori—quality criteria for inclusion and exclusion. They have recommended instead that quality be treated as only one of the many characteristics, or covariates, of a study in "a posteriori analyses" (Cooper, 1998, p. 83). When there is uncertainty or disagreement concerning whether a study meets quality criteria for a research synthesis project, it is better to err on the side of inclusion as this approach tends to offset a greater error by "substituting a discovery process for the predispositions of the synthesist" (Cooper, 1998, p. 84).

The mere fact that a set of qualitative findings does not embody the stated method does not warrant their exclusion. What a hermeneutic analysis is to one reviewer may constitute nothing more than a manifest content analysis to another reviewer. What is methodological confusion, inconsistency, and "impurity" to one reviewer may constitute methodological innovation, eclecticism, and pluralism to another reviewer. Unlike quantitative research, no direct link may be apparent between methods and findings in qualitative research. Not only does the execution of the many methodological approaches constituting qualitative research vary within and across disciplines, but method also functions in qualitative research more to stimulate analysis than to determine or constitute findings (Eakin & Mykhalovskiy, 2003). The rejection of a study that, in the judgment of the reviewer, is misrepresented as a hermeneutic study does not by itself justify the rejection of its findings, if those findings are coherent and well supported by the data presented. A claim to having used a method that is not supported by the content and form of the findings does not by itself leave the findings without empirical support.

The typology derives from our beliefs that: (a) research reports constitute a literary technology mediating between readers/reviewers and writers/researchers; (b) the research synthesis enterprise is both scientific and literary; and (c) readers/reviewers of reports of qualitative studies must, therefore, have research and "literary competence" (Culler, 1980). A competent reader of qualitative research will understand the report as an after-the-fact reconstruction of a study and, therefore, read reports for what they reveal about what was likely done in a study, as opposed to what was claimed or intended. The typology of findings we present here is primarily in the service of achieving that competence as having it will enhance the "utilization value" (Smaling, 2003, pp. 20–21) of qualitative findings and permit more discriminating judgments concerning qualitative research.

THE QUALITY OF QUALITATIVE RESEARCH

Diverse opinions continue to be voiced concerning the right way to conduct the many forms of inquiry referred to as qualitative research. Over the last 20 years, reams of articles and books have been written on the subject of quality in qualitative research, and numerous tools to appraise qualitative research have been promoted (Spencer, Ritchie, Lewis, & Dillon, 2003). Addressing such concepts as reliability and rigor, value and validity, and criteria and credibility, scholars across the practice and social science disciplines have sought to define what a good, valid, and/or trustworthy qualitative study is, to chart the history of and to categorize efforts to accomplish such a definition, and to describe and codify techniques for both ensuring and recognizing good studies (e.g., Devers, 1999; Emden & Sandelowski, 1998, 1999; Engel & Kuzel, 1992; Maxwell, 1992; Seale, 1999; Sparkes, 2001; Whittemore, Chase, & Mandle, 2001).

Yet after all of this effort, no consensus has been reached on quality criteria, or even on whether it is appropriate to try to establish such a consensus. Garratt and Hodkinson (1998) questioned whether there could ever be "preordained" (p. 517) "criteria for selecting research criteria" (p. 515). Sparkes (2001) stated it was a "myth" that qualitative health researchers will ever agree about validity. Kvale (1995) suggested that the quest for quality might itself be an obsession interfering with quality. And Aguinaldo (2004) proposed that discussions of validity are ultimately exercises in power—in rhetoric and representational politics—aimed at legitimating certain ways of knowing and knowledge and de-legitimating others.

The major reason for this lack of consensus is that no "in principle" (Engel & Kuzel, 1992, p. 506) arguments can uniformly address quality in the varieties of practices designated as qualitative research. As Schwandt (2000, p. 190) observed, qualitative research is "home" for a wide variety of scholars across the disciplines who appear to share very little except their general distaste for and distrust of "mainstream" research. Indeed, these scholars are often seriously at odds with each other. Accordingly, it is not surprising that these different communities of qualitative researchers have emphasized different quality criteria. Standards for qualitative research have variously emphasized literary and scientific criteria, methodological rigor and conformity, the real-world significance of the questions asked, the practical value of the findings, and the extent of involvement with, and personal benefit to, research participants (e.g., Emden & Sandelowski, 1998, 1999; Heron, 1996; Lincoln & Reason, 1996; Richardson, 2000a, b; Whittemore, Chase, & Mandle, 2001).

Moving from orientations to quality to the shop floor of research, a key problem with existing tools for appraising qualitative studies is that they confuse the adequacy of a description of something in a report with the appropriateness of something that occurred in the study itself, as represented in the report. A case in point is the sample. Existing criteria frequently do not ask reviewers to differentiate between an informationally adequate description of a sample and a sample adequate to support a claim to informational redundancy. In the first instance, the writer has given either enough or not enough information about the sample to evaluate it. In the second instance, the reader makes a judgment that the sample is or is not large enough to support a claim the writer has made. In the first instance, a judgment is made about adequacy of reporting. In the second instance, a judgment is made about the appropriateness of the reported sample itself (i.e., its size and configuration) to support the findings. In other words, a judgment of reporting adequacy has to be made before a judgment of procedural or interpretive appropriateness can be made. Before readers can make a judgment about anything, writers must have given enough information about it in their reports. A judgment of procedural or interpretive appropriateness (i.e., is it good or valid?) presumes a judgment of reporting adequacy (i.e., is it on the page?).

But the reader must also have an appreciation for the reporting constraints that may have been placed on the writer, such as page limitations and journal and disciplinary conventions concerning what needs to be explicitly said, what can be implied, and what can be omitted. The absence of something in a report does not mean the absence of that thing in the study itself. Moreover, readers themselves will vary in their willingness to accept a reporting absence. While reviewing five studies we had selected for the expert panel in the Metasynthesis Project, one panel member reported that she was most influenced by the absence of information in a report. As she explained it, if a researcher said nothing about method, then method became highly influential in how she viewed the study. Another reviewer suggested a presence/absence calculus in that the presence of findings "with grab" could favorably offset for her the absence of a well-defined problem or method.

Just as the absence of something in a report does not necessarily mean it was absent in the study itself, so too the presence of something in a report does not necessarily mean it was present in the study itself. A writer may have reported that he used phenomenological methods, but the reader—in her judgment of what constitutes phenomenology—finds no discernible evidence of the use of those methods in the findings. A description of a procedure may be judged informationally adequate but informationally and/or procedurally inappropriate. A writer may adequately describe the inter-rater reliability coding technique used to validate study findings, but the reader may judge the rendering of the technique itself as inaccurate and/or the actual use of such techniques as inappropriate to the narrative claims made in a study. In addition, a writer may be forced to discuss matters inappropriate to a qualitative study. The best case in point is the frequent discussion of the so-called limitations of qualitative research, where writers may be forced by peer reviewers or editors to state that their sample was not statistically representative or that their findings are not generalizable. Such statements suggest that a researcher/writer does not understand the purpose of sampling in qualitative research, or the fact that idiographic and analytic generalizations are outcomes of qualitative research. Yet such statements may not be reflective of any error on the part of the researcher.

Even when ostensibly the same criteria are used, reviewers will not use them the same way, agree on whether a study has met them, or, if they agree, have the same reasons for agreeing. Indeed, we recognized from our own and our consultants' efforts to appraise studies how infrequently any one set of criteria for evaluating qualitative studies was used and how much intra-reviewer inconsistency exists (Sandelowski & Barroso, 2003). We all relied on our own personal readings and even "rewritings" of the reports themselves, sometimes assuming an aesthetic stance toward research reports (i.e., responding in terms of our total engagement with a report), other times assuming an efferent stance (i.e., reading a report primarily for the clinically relevant information it provided; Rosenblatt, 1978), and, still other times, assuming a scientific stance (i.e., reading primarily for the validity of the methods used to produce findings).

Accordingly, the typology presented here emphasizes *differences in kind* between qualitative *findings* as presented in research reports, not *differences in quality* between qualitative *studies*. Although differences in kind are not always easy to separate from differences in quality and may even entail them, we do not intend for this typology to be used as a tool for evaluating the scholarly merits of a study, or whether it is "good" enough to be included in a research integration study. A study exemplifying a type, or species, of qualitative findings may be judged as either a high or low quality example of its type. In any event, such a judgment is not the purpose of this typology, which is to make reviewers more discriminating readers of qualitative research reports and to prevent the exclusion of findings important to practice for reasons that do not diminish their importance.

EMPIRICAL/ANALYTICAL VERSUS CONSTRUCTIONIST CONCEPTIONS OF DATA AND FINDINGS

Our typology is based on an empirical/analytical orientation to qualitative research, whereby the results of inquiry are viewed as supported by and, therefore, distinguishable from data. The empirical/analytical orientation is most in line with the research synthesis enterprise as it is conventionally conceived (i.e., as an assimilation or integration of research findings). Data here constitute the evidence for (or ground for belief in the credibility of) research findings. Researcher findings are databased, or composed of what researchers concluded, inferred, or interpreted from the data they collected in a study. Qualitative research findings are, thus, the grounded theories, ethnographies, phenomenologies, and other integrated descriptions or explanations produced from the analysis of data obtained from interviews, observations, documents, and artifacts (Sandelowski & Barroso, 2002). The validity of databased studies is said to depend primarily on the ability of researchers to show that their findings are empirically grounded in the data they collected in those studies. Databased findings ought, therefore, to be readily identifiable and separable from: (a) the data themselves, or the quotations, excerpts from field notes, stories, case histories, and the like that researchers used as evidence for their findings about a target phenomenon; (b) data and findings not about that phenomenon; (c) imported data or findings, or data or findings from other studies to which researchers referred to situate their own findings; (d) analytic procedures, or the coding schemes and data displays researchers used to transform their data into findings; and, (e) researchers' discussions of the meaning, implications, or significance of their findings to research, education, practice, or policy making.

In contrast to the databased view of findings is the data-as-constructed view whereby both data and findings are conceived as indistinguishable from each other, from the participants with whom these data and findings were produced, and from the researchers who decided that some, but not other, things were data. Indeed, the word *finding,* implying that entities can be found, is itself at odds with the idea that everything about the research process is socially constructed. *Data* here is not a word signifying anything plural, or countable as this or that number of instances, but rather a singular body of experience. Following the data-as-constructed line of argument, making something into data is the first stage in the process of data transformation. As Wolcott (1994, pp. 3–4) noted:

> Everything has the potential to be data, but nothing *becomes* (emphasis in original) data without the intervention of a researcher who takes note—and often makes note—of some things to the exclusion of others.

In contrast to the *data collection* in the databased line of argument, where data are commodities to be obtained from people from whom, and via procedures from which, these data are distinguishable, the *data generation* in the data-as-constructed line of argument has no independent existence. Data are never raw but already "constructed entities" (Valsiner, 2000, p. 100). Data generation is inseparable from the: (a) researchers who decide what will become data for their projects; (b) specific and irreplicable encounters between researchers and the people and events that are the subjects and objects of study that together produced those data; and, (c) researchers' interpretations of these subjects and objects of study and, in a reflexive move, of themselves and the research process itself. Neither findings nor any other element of the research process or report can be readily separated from each other, nor should such a separation be attempted.

Following the data-as-constructed line of argument, it is as impossible—and even as nonsensical—to extract *findings* from a poetic, dramatic, or storied presentation of qualitative research as it is to extract them from a poem, play, or novel. Conceiving qualitative findings as evidence is considered as nonsensical as conceiving a poem as evidence. (See chapter 1.) Indeed because data can be construed *as* findings, merely retelling a person's story or providing excerpts from interview data can be construed as the end product of qualitative inquiry. The data-as-constructed view is thus antithetical to the qualitative research synthesis enterprise as it is depicted in this book, which depends on explicitly stated and, therefore, readily identifiable findings constructed by researchers.

Although the data-as-constructed view is antithetical to the qualitative research synthesis enterprise as we portray it here, researchers' use of constructionist orientations to frame their studies is not, so long as their reports contain findings that can be distinguished from the data they generated in their studies. Researchers may simultaneously hold constructionist orientations toward target phenomena and methodology (see chapter 4) and the views that (a) data represent something different from findings and (b) the analysis of those data represent something different from the interpretations deriving from that analysis. Indeed, most qualitative research reports in the practice disciplines embody this orientation, as evident in their authors' use of the experimental/APA style. Our use of the word *constructionist* here is only to (a) signify a view of data, findings, and their relationship to each other different from the conventional databased view, and (b) emphasize that researcher-constructed findings, not the data generated by researchers in their studies, are the primary data in qualitative research synthesis studies. In short, to embark on a qualitative research synthesis project implies that the reviewer holds the empirical/analytical view that "results" exist and that these results are subject to synthesis.

TYPOLOGY OF QUALITATIVE FINDINGS

As shown in Figure 5.1, the typology is an ordinal scale with categories on a continuum of data trans*form*ation. Based on an empirical/analytical view of qualitative research findings, findings are classified according to the degree of researcher transformation of data, from no transformation, to transformations that remain very close to data as given (e.g., a summary of informational contents from a manifest content analysis of data) or move far away from data as given (e.g., a phenomenology of self-transcendence). You will see in Figure 5.1 shaded areas between the points on the continuum. These reflect the usually shady or fuzzy areas between categories, allowing you to classify a set of findings as a borderline rather than a model instance of its kind. The idea is not to force a set of findings into any one category, but rather to use the typology dynamically to contemplate what their content and form reflect about the methodology-in-use.

Indeed, you may decide to refine the typology to accommodate better the studies in your project.

Excluding the *no-finding* category, qualitative findings consist of either surveys (topical or thematic) or syntheses (conceptual/thematic descriptions or interpretive explanations) of the data researchers collected in their studies. As shown in Figure 5.1, survey findings in primary studies lend themselves to survey techniques of integration (i.e., qualitative metasummary; see chapter 6), while synthesized findings in primary studies lend themselves to interpretive techniques of integration (i.e., qualitative metasynthesis; see chapter 7).

Although the typology does not address quality per se, we do propose that no-finding reports (to be described below) do not constitute research and that topical survey reports (also to be described below) are equivocal as qualitative research. But this argument is again to emphasize the differences in kind between research and other kinds of scholarly works, and between qualitative research and research that simply uses qualitative data and/or data collection or analysis techniques commonly perceived as qualitative. We do not propose here that either no-finding or topical survey studies are low-quality works in and of themselves. For us, they simply constitute something other than research or qualitative research and, for those reasons alone, may be subject either to exclusion from the sample of a qualitative research synthesis study or to a posteriori analysis.

Yet we recognize that the judgments involved in proposing such differences in kind may also be seen as judgments about differences in quality. Categorizing a study presented as research as something other than research, or a study presented as qualitative research as something other than qualitative research, can certainly be construed as a judgment about quality and a harsh one at that to researchers seeking the "epistemological credibility" (Thorne, Kirkham, & MacDonald-Emes, 1997, p. 170) and "the rhetorical advantages" (Seale, 2002, p. 659) of naming their work as research or as qualitative research, in particular.

But a key feature of our typology is its emphasis, not on what authors named their analytic and interpretive methods, but rather on the contents and form of what they presented as the findings in their reports of the studies they conducted. A focus on the findings themselves reveals the kind of analytic and interpretive work actually performed, no matter what the research rhetoric. What we found as a result of this focus was that although method might matter in some general sense, the method named in the reports we read often mattered very little to the findings in those reports. Such factors as the presence, amount, and absence of verbal text, metaphoric language, quotes, numbers (e.g., frequencies, means, percents), tables, figures, and other textual and visual displays, revealed more about the methodological orientation of a study than any statements of method in the method sections of reports.

In classifying the findings in the studies you review, you should distinguish between the level of abstraction of analysis and interpretation of data discernible in the findings and the level of abstraction of the phenomena, events, or cases that constitute the subjects/objects of analysis and interpretation. For example, findings about taking antiretroviral medications may seem more concrete and tangible than findings about spirituality simply because spirituality is a phenomenon more difficult to articulate and less tangible than drug use. Yet a set of findings about antiretroviral drug use may actually be more transformed (i.e., interpretively removed from data as given) than a set of findings about spirituality, which may do nothing more than offer a list (or survey) of respondents' definitions of spirituality as they were given to the researcher.

Our typology of findings was developed independently from the typology Margaret Kearney (2001) created but is similar to it; we note these similarities in the description that follows. (Kearney was a member of the Expert Panel for the Qualitative Metasynthesis Project.) But our typology differs from hers in several ways. In contrast to her typology, ours does not assume a "gold standard" (Kearney, 2001, p. 149) in qualitative research, nor does it address "discovery" (p. 146) as a way to classify findings. We see "complexity" as residing primarily in the degree of transformation of data, as opposed to the linking of findings in webs of interaction (p. 146). In addition, while her typology leans toward a view of a priori or, as we call them, imported theoretical frameworks as restricting the evidentiary value of qualitative research for practice, our typology leans toward a view of such frameworks as enhancing the evidentiary value of qualitative research. Finally, while Kearney's typology is primarily intended to be a guide to clinicians in the application of qualitative evidence, our typology is primarily intended to bypass the problem of discrepancies between research claims and research behavior as discernible in a research report. We hope, thereby, to salvage qualitative findings that might be lost to practice because they were excluded from research integration studies only for misrepresenting the method used. Emphasizing the form of findings in addition to their content, the typology is also a basis for matching analysis and synthesis techniques to the actual nature of findings.

No Finding

No-finding reports have no findings in the empirical/analytical meaning of that word whereby findings are distinguished from data. *Findings* consist of the databased and integrated discoveries, judgments, and/or pronouncements researchers offer about the phenomena, events, or cases under investigation. Findings are researchers' interpretations of the data they collected or generated in their studies. *Data* consist of the empirical material (e.g., case descriptions, case histories, quotations, incidents, stories, and the like) researchers offer as evidence for or illustrations of their findings.

The defining feature of no-finding reports is the presentation of uninterpreted data as if they were findings. Apparently subscribing to a databased view of research (as evident in the use of the experimental/APA reporting style), but wanting to satisfy the qualitative imperative to give voice to the voiceless (by ostensibly letting the data speak for themselves), the authors of no-finding reports simply reproduce interview data, case histories, and the like in a reduced form with minimal or no interpretation of those data. In these reports, participants' responses are treated as if they were "places where meanings exist as ready-made" and, therefore, as requiring no "further exploration" by researchers (Nijhof, 1997, p. 175).

The presentation of uninterpreted data may be deliberate, as in certain kinds of oral history and testimonials, alternative renderings of ethnographic findings (Richardson, 2000b), and other forms of "transgressive writing" (Schwalbe, 1995, p. 394). Indeed, for qualitative researchers who view any claims to knowledge as disguised claims to power and who see themselves as speaking for the "underdog" (Jensen & Lauritzen, 2005, p. 63), to put forward an interpretation of others is conceived as an "unethical subversion of the liberatory goal of voicing the voiceless" (Sandelowski, 2004, p. 1377). An example of transgressive writing is the Lather and Smithies (1997) book on HIV-positive women, *Troubling the Angels*. Written specifically to protest, "trouble," and defy conventional academic writing forms, this book presents, at the top half of every page, lengthy excerpts from data derived from focus group interviews with HIV-positive women along with, at the bottom half of each page, a confessional-style author commentary on theory, method, and researcher responses. Interspersed are inserts, boxes, and other forms containing information about HIV infection and cultural images of angels. Although empirical data are presented, the authors chose not to make these or any other data over into findings in a highly self-conscious effort to "get out of the way" (p. xiv) of the women to whom they wished to give voice. Because the book is written in a style wholly and deliberately at odds with the experimental-style research report, it offers no discernible findings in the databased sense. Yet, despite the lack of conventional findings, the book may have value for a research synthesis study by suggesting a metaphor ("angels") that could be used for the qualitative metasynthesis of findings (see chapter 7).

In most qualitative research in the practice disciplines, however, the presentation of uninterpreted data is not intended and is typically the result of mistaking heaped data (Wolcott, 1994, p. 13) for thick description (Geertz, 1973, p. 37). No matter what the authors' intentions, because no-finding reports contain read-only excerpts of data, they have to be excluded from studies aimed at the synthesis of qualitative research findings. Such reports contain no researcher-generated interpretations (or findings in the empirical/analytical sense previously described) that can be integrated with other researcher-generated interpretations.

Topical Survey

More transformed than no-finding reports are reports with findings in the form of topical surveys. Topical surveys are quantitatively-informed inventories of data. The defining features of the topical survey are the reduction of qualitative data in ways that remain close to those data as they were given to the researcher, the nominal use of concepts or themes to organize data, and the nominal use of quotations to illustrate them. Topical surveys feature lists and inventories of topics covered by research participants. This kind of work can be compared to the table of contents of a book (Kearney, 2001) or to a Lands' End catalog. Largely derived from manifest content analyses of individual interview or focus group data, topical surveys emphasize inventories, frequencies, and percentages of research participants stating a topic, or enumerations of the topics themselves. Like a Lands' End catalog, in which merchandise is arranged in surface categories of men's, women's, and children's clothing, data in topical surveys are organized into surface classification systems (e.g., physical, psychological, social, spiritual, or individual, family, community) and they are summarized in brief texts and tables. Like topical anesthesia, topical surveys remain on the surface of words and they treat individual and group interview data as uncomplicated reports of facts and feelings (Sandelowski, 2001). The usual format of the topical survey is to name a topic, briefly define it, and illustrate it with a few examples or quotations.

Because they contain only summaries as opposed to syntheses of data and are, therefore, at best, only borderline examples of qualitative research, you will have to decide whether you want to include them as qualitative research in your qualitative research synthesis study. These studies are valuable, albeit non-categorical descriptive works: that is, works that typically meet neither the probability sampling or psychometric requirements of quantitative surveys, nor the purposeful sampling or interpretive requirements of qualitative research. Favoring inclusion is the fact that the findings in many reports of research designated as qualitative are of this kind and they often contain findings important to practice. Indeed, these were the reports that stimulated the development of qualitative metasummary as a method to integrate the findings contained in them (see chapter 6). But favoring exclusion is the desire to preserve the integrity of "qualitative research" as entailing more than a manifest survey treatment of data.

Thematic Survey

More transformed than the topical survey are findings in the form of thematic surveys. Truer to the interpretive meaning of *theme*, thematic surveys convey a latent pattern or repetition researchers discerned in their data, and a stronger emphasis on qualifying findings as opposed to merely cataloging or enumerating them. (In common usage, *topic* and *theme* are synonymous. In the qualitative research literature, these terms are not used in any consistent way. See DeSantis & Ugarriza, 2000 and Fredericks & Miller, 1997.)

Thematic survey findings reveal a discernible effort to move away from merely listing topics (or the subjects brought up by research participants in interviews) toward describing themes (or the patterned responses researchers themselves discerned in the topics raised). Thematic survey findings move farther way from the data as given to researchers and further into those data to capture more of the subtleties of experience. Thematic surveys are more penetrating or nuanced treatments of data, labeled and organized by the in vivo (i.e., everyday) language of research participants, or by concepts imported from empirical or theoretical literature (e.g., *passing* and *covering* in the stigma literature, *attachment* and *loss* in the bereavement literature). Although thematic surveys offer more verbal text than topical surveys, the mere presence of more words as opposed to numbers is not what separates a thematic from a topical survey. Rather, what distinguishes the one from the other is the extent to which researchers interpretively penetrated the data they obtained, or detailed the experiences these data represented.

An example of a report with findings in the form of a thematic survey is the Siegel & Schrimshaw (2001) study (featured in chapter 4), which offers a fine-grained description of the reasons and justifications a group of HIV-positive women gave for having children.

Conceptual/Thematic Description

More transformed than thematic surveys are findings rendered in the form of one or more concepts or themes either developed in situ (i.e., invented by the researcher from the data collected in a study), or imported from theoretical or empirical literature outside the study. Analogous to each other in degree of interpretive transformation, *conceptual descrip-tion* refers to theoretical renderings of phenomena, events, or cases commonly associated with the social sciences and/or grounded theory work, while *thematic description* refers to narrative, phenomenological, or discursive renderings of experience. We use the words *concept* and *theme* here, as opposed to *topic*, to convey researchers' efforts to describe a latent, as opposed to manifest, pattern in the data.

Conceptual/thematic descriptions move beyond surveying the topical or thematic landscape of data. In contrast to thematic surveys, in which in situ or imported concepts or themes are used largely to organize data and the presentation of findings, in conceptual or thematic descriptions, concepts or themes are used to reframe a phenomenon, event, or case. Whereas topical and thematic surveys are characterized by the nominal use of concepts or themes to label and order portions of data, conceptual/thematic descriptions are characterized by the interpretive use of concepts or themes to integrate and, thereby, recast portions of data. In conceptual/thematic descriptions, concepts are actually used conceptually and themes are actually used thematically. Findings in this form serve not only as a reasonable way to group and present data, but also to illuminate experience and/or, if imported, to extend the theoretical or other intellectual tradition from which they were derived.

An example of findings in the form of a conceptual description is the Ingram & Hutchinson (2000) report, in which the concept of the "double bind" is imported to integrate data. An example of findings in the form of a thematic description is the Vantine (2000) report, in which "paradox" is presented as the thematic thread linking data.

Interpretive Explanation

The most transformed of qualitative findings is the interpretive explanation, or the grounded theories, ethnographies, or otherwise fully integrated explanations of phenomena, events, or cases considered the quintessence of qualitative research. In contrast to findings that consist of surveys of topics and themes, or of conceptual/thematic treatments of segments of data representing one or more elements of an experience, interpretive explanations offer a coherent model, or single thesis or line of argument, which addresses causality or the fundamental nature of events or experiences. These explanations attend to relevant variations in both sample and data, and come to a point or take a specific view in rendering target phenomena. Because findings in this category emphasize explanation and variation, they are most akin to findings Kearney (2001) described as "dense explanatory description" (p. 149), with features of her "shared pathway" and "depiction of experiential variation" categories (p. 148).

Whereas a topical or thematic survey might consist of a list, or more detailed description, of a set of concerns HIV-positive women expressed, and a conceptual description, a reframing of these concerns as rationalizations, an interpretive explanation will consist of an interpretive accounting of how each of these concerns was a condition for distinctively different defensive strategies, only some of which succeeded in allaying those concerns. Although the most complex of the types of findings featured here, interpretive explanations are the easiest to identify and extract precisely because they are the most integrated.

An example of findings in the form of an interpretive explanation is the Grove, Kelly, & Liu (1997) report, in which they argue for the greater capacity of women deemed to be "nice girls" to offset the negative social effects of HIV infection.

REFERENCES

Aguinaldo, J. P. (2004). Rethinking validity in qualitative research from a social constructionist perspective: From "Is this valid research?" to "What is this research valid for?" *The Qualitative Report, 9(1)*, 127–136. Retrieved December 1, 2004, from www.nova.edu/ssss/QR/QR9-1/aguinaldo.pdf

Barbour, R. S. (2001). Checklists for improving rigor in qualitative research: A case of the tail wagging the dog? *British Medical Journal, 322*, 1115–1117.

Conn, V. S., & Rantz, M. J. (2003). Research methods: Managing primary study quality in meta-analyses. *Research in Nursing & Health, 26*, 322–333.

Cooper, H. (1998). *Synthesizing research: A guide for literature reviews* (3rd ed.). Thousand Oaks, CA: Sage.

Culler, J. (1980). Literary competence. In J. Tompkins (Ed.), *Reader-response criticism: From formalism to post-structuralism* (pp. 101–117). Baltimore: Johns Hopkins University Press.

DeSantis, L., & Ugarriza, D. N. (2000). The concept of theme as used in qualitative nursing research. *Western Journal of Nursing Research, 22*, 351–372.

Devers, K. J. (1999). How will we know "good" qualitative research when we see it? Beginning the dialogue in health services research. *HSR: Health Services Research, 34*, 1153–1188.

Eakin, J. M., & Mykhalovskiy, E. (2003). Reframing the evaluation of qualitative health research: Reflections on a review of appraisal guidelines on the health sciences. *Journal of Evaluation in Clinical Practice, 9*, 187–194.

Emden, C., & Sandelowski, M. (1998). The good, the bad, and the relative, part 1: Conceptions of goodness in qualitative research. *International Journal of Nursing Practice, 4*, 206–212.

Emden, C., & Sandelowski, M. (1999). The good, the bad, and the relative, part 2: Goodness and the criterion problem in qualitative research. *International Journal of Nursing Practice, 5*, 2–7.

Engel, J. D., & Kuzel, A. J. (1992). On the idea of what constitutes good qualitative inquiry. *Qualitative Health Research, 2*, 504–510.

Fredericks, M., & Miller, S. I. (1997). Some brief notes on the "unfinished business" of qualitative inquiry. *Quality & Quantity, 31,* 1–13.

Garratt, D., & Hodkinson, P. (1998). Can there be criteria for selecting research criteria? A hermeneutical analysis of an inescapable dilemma. *Qualitative Inquiry, 4,* 515–539.

Geertz, C. (1973). Thick description: Toward an interpretive theory of culture. In C. Geertz, *The interpretation of cultures: Selected essays* (pp. 37–126). New York: Basic Books.

Glass, G. V. (2000). *Meta-analysis at 25.* Retrieved August 19, 2003, from http://glass.ed.asu.edu/gene/papers/meta25.html

Grove, K. A., Kelly, D. P., & Liu, J. (1997). "But nice girls don't get it": Women, symbolic capital, and the social construction of AIDS. *Journal of Contemporary Ethnography, 26,* 317–337.

Heron, J. (1996). Quality as primacy of the practical. *Qualitative Inquiry, 2,* 41–56.

Ingram, D., & Hutchinson, S. A. (2000). Double binds and the reproductive and mothering experiences of HIV-positive women. *Qualitative Health Research, 10,* 117–132.

Jensen, C., & Lauritsen, P. (2005). Qualitative research as partial connection: Bypassing the power-knowledge nexus. *Qualitative Research, 5,* 59–77.

Kaplan, A. (1964). *The conduct of inquiry: Methodology for behavioral science.* San Francisco: Chandler.

Kearney, M. H. (2001). Levels and applications of qualitative research evidence. *Research in Nursing & Health, 24,* 145–153.

Kvale, S. (1995). The social construction of validity. *Qualitative Inquiry, 1,* 19–40.

Lather, P., & Smithies, C. (1997). *Troubling the angels: Women living with HIV/AIDS.* Boulder, CO: Westview Press.

Lincoln, Y. S., & Reason, P. (Eds.). (1996). Quality in human inquiry (Entire issue). *Qualitative Inquiry, 2(1).*

Maxwell, J. A. (1992). Understanding and validity in qualitative research. *Harvard Educational Review, 62,* 279–300.

Nijhof, G. (1997). "Response work": Approaching answers to open interviews as readings. *Qualitative Inquiry, 3,* 169–187.

Richardson, L. (2000a). Evaluating ethnography. *Qualitative Inquiry, 6,* 253–255.

Richardson, L. (2000b). Writing: A method of inquiry. In N. K. Denzin & Y. S. Lincoln (Eds.), *Handbook of qualitative research* (2nd ed., pp. 923–948). Thousand Oaks, CA: Sage.

Rosenblatt, L. M. (1978). *The reader, the text, the poem: The transactional theory of the literary work.* Carbondale: Southern Illinois University Press.

Sandelowski, M. (2001). Reembodying qualitative inquiry. *Qualitative Health Research, 12,* 104–115.

Sandelowski, M. (2004). Using qualitative research. *Qualitative Health Research, 14,* 1366–1386.

Sandelowski, M., & Barroso, J. (2002). Finding the findings in qualitative studies. *Journal of Nursing Scholarship, 34,* 213–219.

Sandelowski, M., & Barroso, J. (2003). Classifying the findings in qualitative studies. *Qualitative Health Research, 7,* 905–923.

Schwalbe, M. (1995). The responsibilities of sociological poets. *Qualitative Sociology, 18,* 393–413.

Schwandt, T. A. (2000). Three epistemological stances for qualitative inquiry: Interpretivism, hermeneutics, and social constructionism. In N. K. Denzin & Y. S. Lincoln (Eds.), *Handbook of qualitative research* (2nd ed., pp. 189–213). Thousand Oaks, CA: Sage.

Seale, C. (1999). *The quality of qualitative research.* London: Sage.

Seale, C. (2002). Computer-assisted analysis of qualitative interview data. In J. F. Gubrium & J. A. Holstein (Eds.), *Handbook of interview research* (pp. 651–670). Thousand Oaks, CA: Sage.

Siegel, K., & Schrimshaw, E. W. (2001). Reasons and justifications for considering pregnancy among women living with HIV/AIDS. *Psychology of Women Quarterly, 25,* 112–123.

Slavin, R. E. (1995). Best evidence synthesis: An intelligent alternative to meta-analysis. *Journal of Clinical Epidemiology, 48,* 9–18.

Smaling, A. (2003). Inductive, analogical, and communicative generalization. *International Journal of Qualitative Methods, 2(1).* Article 5. Retrieved September 22, 2003, from http://www.ualberta.ca/~ijqm/backissues/2_1/html/smaling.html

Sparkes, A. C. (2001). Myth 94: Qualitative health researchers will agree about validity. *Qualitative Health Research, 11,* 538–552.

Spencer, L., Ritchie, J., Lewis, J., & Dillon, L. (2003). *Quality in qualitative evaluation: A framework for assessing research evidence.* London: Government Chief Social Researcher's Office (Retrieved March 4, 2004, from http://www.policyhub.gov.uk/docs/qqe_rep.pdf).

Thorne, S. Kirkham, S. R., & MacDonald-Emes, J. (1997). Interpretive description: A noncategorical qualitative alternative for developing nursing knowledge. *Research in Nursing & Health, 20,* 169–177.

Valsiner, J. (2000). Data as representations: Contextualizing qualitative and quantitative research strategies. *Social Science Information, 39,* 99–113.

Vantine, H. S. (2000). *Terminating a wanted pregnancy after the discovery of possible fetal abnormalities: An existential phenomenological study of making and living with the decision.* Unpublished doctoral dissertation, Duquesne University, Pittsburgh, PA.

Whittemore, R., Chase, S. K., & Mandle, C. L. (2001). Validity in qualitative research. *Qualitative Health Research, 11,* 522–537.

Wolcott, H. F. (1994). *Transforming qualitative data: Description, analysis, and interpretation.* Thousand Oaks, CA: Sage.

CHAPTER SIX

Synthesizing Qualitative Research Findings:
Qualitative Metasummary

Now that you know each report in your study about as well as the back of your hand, and have classified the findings, you are ready to consider approaches to integrating the findings across reports. You will recall that qualitative metasummary and qualitative metasynthesis are the two approaches to qualitative research synthesis we are featuring in this book.

Qualitative metasummary (the subject of this chapter) is a quantitatively oriented aggregation of qualitative findings that are themselves topical or thematic summaries or surveys of data. Metasummaries address the manifest content in findings across reports in a target domain of research and reflect a quantitative logic: to discern the frequency of each finding and to find in higher frequency findings the evidence of replication foundational to validity in quantitative research and to the claim of having discovered a pattern or theme (Sandelowski, 2001), or "preponderance of evidence" (Thorne, Jensen, Kearney, Noblit, & Sandelowski, 2004, p. 1362), in qualitative research. Qualitative metasummaries can serve as end points of research synthesis studies containing largely survey findings, or as an empirical foundation for, or bridge to, qualitative metasynthesis, preparing survey findings for metasynthesis and optimizing the validity of the integration produced.

Qualitative metasynthesis (the subject of chapter 7) is an interpretive integration of qualitative findings that are themselves interpretive syntheses of data, including the phenomenologies, ethnographies, grounded theories, and other integrated and coherent descriptions or explanations of phenomena, events, or cases that are the hallmarks of qualitative research. Metasyntheses are integrations that are more than summaries in that they offer novel interpretations of findings. These interpretations will not be found in any one research report, but rather are derived from taking all of the reports in a sample as a whole. Metasyntheses offer a coherent description or explanation of a target event or experience, instead of a summary view of unlinked features of that event or experience. Such interpretive integrations require researchers to piece the individual syntheses constituting the findings in individual research reports together to craft one or more metasyntheses. In contrast to qualitative metasummary, which emphasizes reportage and a surface penetration of research findings, qualitative metasynthesis emphasizes the more penetrating interpretive acts of reading into and between the lines and overreading (Poirier & Ayres, 1997). In qualitative metasyntheses, language is viewed as a structure or artifact of culture that must itself be interpreted, not merely as a vehicle of communication. Their validity does not reside in a replication logic, but rather in an interpretive logic, whereby findings are reframed, and in the craftsmanship exhibited in the final product.

QUALITATIVE METASUMMARY

Qualitative metasummary techniques include: (a) extracting findings, separating them from other elements of the research report; (b) editing findings to make them accessible to any reader; (c) grouping findings in common topical domains; (d) abstracting findings; and (e) calculating manifest frequency and intensity effect sizes.

Extracting Findings

This phase entails distinguishing the specific findings you want to integrate from all other elements in the research reports containing those findings. Recall that we are defining *findings* here as consisting of researchers' interpretations of the interview, observation, and other data they collected or generated in their studies.

Defining the Target Findings

To begin the extraction process, you must have a working definition of the findings that interest you. This definition will help you identify what material to extract and maintain consistency in the extraction process. For example, when our research purpose was to explore the experience of motherhood in HIV-positive women, we defined *motherhood finding* as any researcher interpretation specifically addressing women's decisions to become mothers and the experiences of becoming or being mothers to, or of having or caring for, minor children.

As you work, you will likely expand your definition (and, therefore, extract more material) or further limit your definition (and, therefore, extract less material). Every time you alter your working definition, you must return to those reports from which you extracted material under the previous definition and extract findings under the new definition. Be careful that the findings you are extracting are truly about your target area. For example, in several reports in our HIV sample, researchers used the word *mother* as a synonym for *woman,* but offered no finding specific to motherhood.

Separating Findings

The specific research findings you are seeking must be separated in every relevant report from:

1. Presentations of data, or the quotations, incidents, stories, and case histories researchers used to provide evidence for their findings;
2. Data and findings not about the target area;
3. Imported findings, or findings from other studies to which researchers referred;
4. Analytic procedures, or descriptions of the coding schemes, data displays, and the like researchers used to produce their findings; and from
5. Researchers' discussions of the meaning, implications, or significance of their findings to research, education, practice, or policy making.

As you are deciding what material to extract, be sure to:

6. Treat each report as one unit of analysis, no matter what the page length (which is subject to a host of publication constraints) or the size of the sample (which is appropriately variable in qualitative research);
7. Link findings to sample variations or subgroups, if this can be discerned;
8. Link findings to varying conditions or circumstances, if this can be discerned;
9. Determine whether the quotations or incidents researchers offer support their interpretations;
10. Determine whether findings sufficiently differentiate among (a) participants' own thoughts, feelings, or behaviors; (b) their understandings of other peoples' thoughts, feelings, or behaviors;

and (c) their accounts of hypothetical instances of, or prescriptions for, thoughts, feelings, or behaviors; and
11. Note whether findings were derived from your target subjects
themselves or from proxies for them.

We have itemized these distinctions to help you clarify your focus,
notice other distinctions that may be relevant to the body of literature addressed in your study, and optimize the descriptive and interpretive validity of your findings (see chapter 8). For example, quotations are
typically used as evidence in support of findings, but they may not fit the
conclusions drawn or illustrate the points intended by the author. As they
are only extracts from a larger data set, the quotations appearing in reports may suggest an entirely different line of interpretation or detract
from a given interpretation because they contain too much or too little information, or because they are not appropriately staged (Sandelowski,
1994). Findings may consist of combinations of descriptions (e.g., what
happened), prescriptions (e.g., what ought to have happened), and prob-
abilities (e.g., what might have happened), or of what a group of participants themselves felt or did and of what they surmised or observed others
in their situation felt or did, or ought to feel or do. Interview data are
messy and it is the messiness of these data that makes qualitative analysis
and, therefore, qualitative research synthesis so challenging. In addition,
researchers often do not collect data in ways that make these distinctions
or attend to them in their analyses. Accordingly, concluding that, for
example, participants routinely avoided social interaction may not be as
accurate as concluding that they routinely observed that other people in
their circumstances should avoid it. After tracking the sources of data
in each report, you must decide whether your research purpose mandates inclusion of findings derived only from participants themselves
(e.g., HIV-positive women), or derived both from and about them (e.g.,
interviews with HIV-positive women, and interviews with their children,
partners, and nurses, and information from medical records). Accordingly,
if your research purpose is to ascertain a particular group of participants'
points of view, you may decide to exclude findings that are not directly
from the target participants.

Because writers of qualitative research reports often amend the experimental-style format to include references to other literature in the
results section (as opposed to reserving them for the discussion section),
distinguishing in situ findings (i.e., findings generated from the data collected within the confines of a study) from other material in a report can
be hard to do. A case in point is Weitz's (1993) informative article on the
experiences of women living with HIV infection, which was derived
from her book on *Life With AIDS* (1991) in men and women. We found
it difficult to discern which of her findings were in fact derived from the

interviews in her study, or from other studies. For example, the first statement in the section called "children's and women's lives" concerning HIV-positive mothers that might be construed as a finding was:

> Both having and not having children can create problems for persons with HIV disease. This issue is far more salient for women than for men, however, because women are taught from childhood to find fulfillment and self-worth primarily through childrearing and because women more often than men find themselves single parents (Weitz, 1993, p. 112).

This statement is followed, not by any presentation of interview data, but rather by three paragraphs that, like the preceding one, present general information about HIV-positive women derived from sources other than the women interviewed. The first reference in this section to any woman actually interviewed in her study is when Weitz reported that half of the childless women regarded their childlessness as a major source of grief in their lives, and then quoted one woman as evidence for this conclusion. Contributing to the difficulty in discerning the in situ findings in this report are numerous statements like this one:

> Those women who already have children face a different set of problems. . . . The women may enjoy a new closeness with their children, as they discover how much they mean to each other and begin to spend more time together (Weitz, 1993, p. 113).

These sentences are written in the generalizing present tense ("women who already have children face . . .") and in hypothetical terms ("women may enjoy . . ."). The problem here is the reader cannot be sure if the women referred to were the women in the study. Although Weitz used quotations from the women she interviewed, they seem to function more as evidence for the generalizations derived from studies other than her own. These statements illustrate how even ostensibly insignificant features of grammar and syntax can obscure the source of findings and, thereby, compel reviewers to choose whether to include them as findings. In the examples here, reviewers must decide whether to read "women who already have children face . . ." as "the women who already had children faced . . ." and to read "women may enjoy . . ." as "the women enjoyed . . ." Reviewers may also decide to contact researchers themselves to clarify their findings.

Editing Findings

Once you have finished extracting findings, you should edit them to make them as accessible as possible to any reader. This entails staying as close as possible to the words of researchers/authors and preserving their intentions while clarifying them for readers who will not have read the report in which they appear. Usually only minor editing is required to transform what researchers/authors presented as findings into complete sentences readers can understand. The last section of Table 4.1 in chapter 4 shows the results of the extraction and editing processes for the research report featured there. Please visit the supplement to chapter 6 at http://www.unc.edu/~msandelo/handbook/site/chapter6.html to see a more dynamic presentation of the extraction and editing processes.

Table 6.1 shows the results of the extraction and editing processes applied to 4 of the 56 reports of qualitative studies conducted with HIV-positive women. You will note that two of the reports are of studies that had as their research purposes the exploration of motherhood, while two of the reports are of studies with other research purposes (i.e., living with HIV and disclosure). This underscores the evolving nature of qualitative research, whereby findings are produced on topics not anticipated. Thirty-three of the 56 research reports of studies with findings pertaining to motherhood had research purposes other than the exploration of motherhood. (Had we restricted our study of motherhood only to reports of studies that had as their research purposes the exploration of some aspect of motherhood, we would have unknowingly eliminated over half of the reports of studies with motherhood findings. See chapter 3.)

Grouping Findings

After you have extracted and edited all of the findings that address your research purpose, you will be ready to group findings that appear to be about the same topic. You will have gained a sense of the range of topics covered in the findings from having worked so closely with each report in your study. Here is an example of findings from three reports that all pertain to the topic of mothers disclosing their HIV status to children. The findings from the first study indicate that:

- Mothers universally struggle with whether to disclose their HIV diagnosis to young children.
- Most mothers have decided against disclosure to children.
- A reason for not disclosing is the perceived inability of young children to understand or deal with impending maternal death.
- The decision not to disclose to children means that mothers will not have to spend time and energy soothing their worries.
- The results of decisions about disclosure have ramifications.
- Disclosure to a young child may lead to unwanted disclosure to neighbors, friends, and acquaintances.

The findings from the second study indicate that:

- Mothers were concerned about the ability of children to keep HIV secret.
- Mothers were concerned about children's reaction to disclosure.
- Mothers were concerned about children's reaction to them after disclosure.
- Maternal strategies used to combat uncertainty over disclosure of HIV to child included not telling, timing the disclosure, and selective disclosure.

The findings from the third study indicate that:

- Mothers demonstrated a concern that by disclosing their HIV status they might be transferring the potential stigmatization associated with HIV/AIDS to their children.
- Some women reported that telling their HIV status to their children face to face was one of the most difficult parts of the disease process.

Grouping findings according to their topical similarity will allow you to see how findings within each topical group are related to each other. You will see whether findings about the same event or experience (a) replicate or confirm, (b) extend, or (c) refute each other. An example of *replication* or *confirmation* is when a specified number of reports all indicate that HIV-positive women found it hard to disclose their HIV status to their children. An example of *extension* is when a specified number of reports focus on HIV-positive women's patterns of disclosure, but some focus on patterns of disclosure to children, while others emphasize patterns of disclosure to partners, relatives, friends, and coworkers. What is extended in this example is information about patterns of disclosure to different targets of disclosure. What is also extended is information about relationships with children. Accordingly, these findings might initially or subsequently be grouped in at least three ways: as all about disclosure, as all about children, or as all about disclosing maternal HIV status to children.

An example of refutation is when one set of findings indicates that religion influenced the decision-making process of couples receiving positive fetal diagnoses, while another set indicates that religion had no influence. The finding in one study indicates that:

- Although a large number of the participants in this study were Catholic, religion did not seem to play a major role in their decision.

The finding on the same topic (i.e., influence of religion on decision making) in another study indicates that:

- Women with strong religious affiliations, strong kinship or other communitarian social support, or strong reasons anchored in their reproductive histories are most likely to decide against the biomedical information amniocentesis brings as a basis for accepting or rejecting a pregnancy.
- Women with Catholic backgrounds seemed especially susceptible to guilt.

After further analysis of these and other reports, you may decide that these findings do not refute, but rather extend each other by capturing different circumstances (e.g., strong versus weak religious affiliations, Catholic versus other religions), or require further delineation in future research projects.

Grouping entails placing findings on the same topic together, even when they contradict each other within the same report or across reports. The grouping process entails putting findings about the *same topic* (e.g., disclosure of HIV status) together, not putting findings that say the *same thing* about the same topic together (e.g., that religion played a major role in couples' decision making following positive fetal diagnosis). Seeing *all* the findings pertaining to *one* topic together will help you preserve the integrity and complexity of the findings as given in the research reports and, thereby, optimize the validity of the integration process. Grouping findings about the same topic will allow you to see the different relationships that exist among findings (i.e., whether they say the same thing about the same topic, or different and even contradictory things about the same topic). Because you are the judge of what is the same or different and of what is a confirmation, extension, or refutation (i.e., *sameness, difference, confirmation, extension,* and *refutation* are themselves interpretations), and because these judgments are likely to change as you move deeper into the analysis of findings, you should track the course of your judgments. The validity of your integration study resides in the documentation of these turns in judgments.

Grouping findings in common topical areas will also enable you to see whether findings in different topical areas complement each other. An example of a complementary relationship in the HIV reports we reviewed is that stigma was a key component of findings pertaining to motherhood (topic A), while motherhood was a key component of findings pertaining to stigma (topic B). After further analysis of findings pertaining to both motherhood and stigma, we proposed a conceptual relationship between them whereby HIV-related stigma intensified the negative effects of motherhood, but motherhood both intensified and mitigated the negative effects of HIV-related stigma.

Table 6.2 shows another example of the grouping process applied to five reports. Please visit the supplement to chapter 6 at http://www.unc.edu/~msandelo/handbook/site/chapter6.html to see a more dynamic presentation of the grouping process.

Abstracting Findings

In the abstraction process, you will further reduce the many statements of findings you extracted, edited, and grouped into more parsimonious renderings of them. Create files (in whatever text management system you prefer) in which you can see all topically similar findings together. Working in each file, move back and forth between the edited statements of topically similar extracted findings and your developing statements of abstracted findings until you have a set of statements that concisely but comprehensively captures the content of all the findings and preserves the context in which they appeared. To accomplish this, you should:

1. eliminate redundancies in the findings;
2. refine statements to be inclusive of the ideas researchers conveyed in their findings; and
3. preserve the contradictions and ambiguities in the findings.

Once you have a complete set of abstracted findings, assign each one to those reports in your study that contain findings captured in each abstraction. Box 6.1 shows the results of the abstraction process applied to findings pertaining to motherhood in HIV-positive women. (The numbers here simply indicate findings; they have no other meaning.) Sixty-seven statements of findings were produced from approximately 2,000 statements of extracted findings from 56 reports.

Calculating Manifest Frequency and Intensity Effect Sizes

To extract more meaning from, and assess the magnitude of, the abstracted findings, you can calculate their effect sizes (Onwuegbuzie, 2003; Onwuegbuzie & Teddlie, 2003). Commonly associated with quantitative meta-analysis, the term *effect size* refers generically to indices of the magnitude of a treatment effect. Although qualitative studies typically do not address treatments, they do address patterns and themes, which inherently imply a frequency of occurrence of an event sufficient to constitute a pattern or theme. The calculation of effect sizes is a way to unite the empirical precision of quantitative research with the descriptive precision of qualitative research. The calculation of effect sizes constitutes a quantitative transformation of qualitative data in the service of extracting more meaning from those data and verifying the presence of a pattern or theme. Effect sizes in qualitative studies are both a means to ensure that findings are neither over- nor underweighted, and they can serve as an empirical basis for qualitative metasynthesis.

Tables 6.3 and 6.4 show frequency and intensity effect sizes of the findings pertaining to motherhood. The inter-study matrix shown in Table 6.3 organizes reports by the abstracted findings. The intra-study matrix shown in Table 6.4 organizes findings by the reports.

Use the inter-study matrix to calculate the *manifest frequency effect size* of each abstracted finding. Take the number of reports containing a finding minus the number of duplicate reports containing that finding and divide this number by the total number of reports containing this finding minus the number of duplicate reports. For example, the frequency effect size of 57% (rounded-off number) of the first finding shown in Table 6.3 was derived by dividing 29 (or the number of reports with this finding minus the number of reports from the same study with common samples containing the same finding) by 51 (the number of total reports in the sample minus the number of reports from the same study with common samples containing the same finding).

Use the intra-study matrix to calculate the *manifest intensity effect size,* or concentration of findings in each report. Take the number of findings in each study and divide this by the total number of findings across all reports. For example, the intensity effect size of 34% in the first report shown in Table 6.4 was derived by dividing 23 (the number of findings contained in the report) by 67 (the total number of findings across reports). Publication venues with fewer space restrictions than print journals, such as dissertations, books, and on line journals, will typically have greater intensity effect sizes. Because of fewer space restrictions, these kinds of publications will also add to the number of findings with weaker frequency effect sizes. Although less frequent, these findings may either clarify the findings in more space-restricted journal articles, or provide direction for the more penetrating analyses associated with qualitative metasyntheses. Intensity effect sizes will also reveal the extent to which any one report contains the findings across all reports in your study. As a result of calculating intensity effect sizes, you will see that one or two works can encompass most of the key findings in a target area. But you can only ascertain this after you have extracted the findings from all the reports in your study.

The move from study report to effect sizes requires you to make a series of judgment calls, which you will have to articulate, defend, and consistently apply, concerning which reports will be used, what material will be extracted as findings, and how findings were transformed in the process of abstraction. By themselves, effect size numbers have no meaning. They acquire their meaning only in relation to each other as they are intended to assess the relative frequency of abstracted findings across reports and concentration of abstracted findings within each report.

Use of Qualitative Metasummary With Synthesized Findings

Although we developed qualitative metasummary to accommodate reports with survey findings, it should be used also to extract the statements of findings encompassed in reports with synthesized findings, or findings in the form of conceptual/thematic descriptions or interpretive explanations. These conceptual syntheses are shown in Box 6.1 as findings 63–67. For example, the key finding in the Ingram (1996) and Ingram and Hutchinson (1999, 2000) reports is that the double bind of motherhood for HIV-positive women led to their practice of defensive motherhood. But we also extracted all the statements of findings—in their unlinked state—which contributed to this grounded theory, as shown in Table 6.5. This process allows the statements contributing to the intra-report syntheses of data into conceptual/thematic descriptions and interpretive explanations to be combined with the unlinked statements that characterize the topical and thematic survey findings (see chapter 5). This process is also necessary for the reciprocal translation and synthesis of these concepts we describe in chapter 7, as it allows you to determine whether and how they can be translated into each other.

In a similar vein, the key finding in the Grove, Kelly, and Liu (1997) study is that HIV-positive women who possess "symbolic capital" (i.e., white, heterosexual, married, educated, and/or middle class) are better able to protect their moral identities. Women with symbolic capital can draw on the cultural dichotomy between us (i.e., "nice girls") and them (i.e., "bad girls"), thereby eliciting sympathy but reproducing the idea of "innocent" as opposed to "guilty" victims of HIV infection. Although being seen as a "nice girl" allows such women to escape some of the negative social effects of HIV infection, such profiling may lead to delayed diagnosis. Thus having symbolic capital is a two-edged sword: destigmatizing but life-threatening. Table 6.6 shows the statements of findings supporting this interpretive explanation.

A Posteriori Analyses of Noise in Abstracted Findings

In chapter 4, we advised you to consider the extent to which the "noise" in a study, or its methodological flaws, detracts from its "signal," or potential value of study findings for practice (Edwards, Elwyn, Hood, & Rollnick,

2000; Edwards, Russell, & Stott, 1998). Here we advise you to determine the extent to which findings you judged to be "noisy" contribute to each one of your abstracted findings. This is an example of the a posteriori analysis leading scholars in the research integration field recommend in lieu of the a priori exclusion of studies for reasons of methodological quality. You may wish to calculate effect sizes with and without the reports you judged to be of questionable value to determine whether the relative magnitude of each finding would dramatically change. You might find, as a result, that one or more of your abstracted findings is almost wholly derived from such studies and, therefore, treat these findings with caution, or exclude. Note here that you are excluding the abstracted findings in question, not necessarily the entire reports from which they were derived. "Noisy" reports may still be retained if they do not constitute the only basis for an abstracted finding.

BOX 6.1 Abstracted Findings Pertaining to Motherhood in HIV-Positive Women Arranged in Topical Groups

Generally positive experiences with motherhood

1. Children were the main reasons to live, fight, get off drugs, care for oneself, and avoid risky behaviors.
2. Whether their children were in or out of their care or custody, being a mother was central to women's lives: a source of self-esteem, strength, normalcy, inspiration, pride, hope, joy, sense of well-being, & sense of self as a whole woman.
3. Children were important sources of physical, practical, emotional, and social support, and unconditional love to their mothers, buffering the negative effects of HIV.
4. HIV had a positive impact on mothering, especially in drug-abusing women and women living with HIV for a longer time.
5. Mothers reported strong physical and psychological attachments to their children, and intensification of the maternal role.
6. Mothering or having children had a positive influence on coping with and symptoms of HIV.
7. Mothers viewed children as their legacy, final acts of creation, rescuers, saviors, and fulfillers of their unfulfilled dreams.

Generally negative experiences with motherhood

8. Mothers worried about the negative impact of maternal HIV (the illness itself and/or its stigma) on their children, including their negative reactions to it and others' negative reactions to their children.
9. The combination of motherhood and HIV was physically demanding.
10. Maternity/life was often the context for HIV diagnosis/death in women.
11. Often the sole caregivers, mothers reported concerns, frustrations, and difficulties disciplining children.
12. Mothers, especially those who had abused drugs or were ill, struggled to establish, maintain, and/or preserve maternal identity while children were out of their care, during illness, and after maternal death.
13. Motherhood or having children had a negative impact on the symptoms and stresses of HIV.

Stigma & disclosure

14. Mothers struggled with whether to disclose their HIV to their children, worried about the effects of disclosure on child and maternal welfare and the maternal-child relationship, and engaged in strategies to disclose or to delay or avoid disclosing their HIV status to their children.
15. Women with children were subject to the triple stigmatization (of drug abuse, promiscuity, and infecting the innocent), and reported stigmatization attributed to HIV infection.
16. Mothers reported that children had varying initial and subsequent reactions to disclosure, including shock, recognition of something they already suspected, concern, sadness, anger, and desire for more information.
17. Rates of disclosure varied by child's age, mother's stage of illness, and custody, with healthier mothers tending not to disclose to younger children or children not in their care.

18. Most mothers who disclosed to children did not regret it and reported closer relations with children.
19. Reasons for disclosing to children included educating children, maintaining honest relations, preempting others disclosing, showing children they were still healthy.
20. Reasons for not disclosing to children included the belief that children were too young or immature to understand; and concerns about the negative impact on children, sequelae of child's then disclosing, the undermining of renewed relations with children, and children's exposure to other losses.
21. By telling others about their HIV, mothers garnered support for themselves and their children, protected others from HIV, but risked more disclosure, rejection, and exposing loved ones to pain.
22. By not telling others, mothers protected themselves and their children from the threat of disclosure, but cut themselves and their children off from sources of support, and left their families and friends unprepared to deal with their impending death.

Mothering the HIV– child vs. HIV+ child
23. Mothers wanted and acted to protect all their children.
24. Mothers had special concerns about, hopes for, and were consumed with the health, illness care, future, and placement of HIV+ children.
25. Mothers reported instances, or worried about the negative effects, of HIV– child role reversal, or had adult expectations of their assuming a mother or caretaking role.
26. Mother-child relations changed with the progress of maternal or child HIV disease.
27. Sick mothers cared for sick children, the care HIV+ mothers of HIV+ children give them detracted from their own health and the care of HIV– children.
28. Maternal attention and attachment, mother-child relations, and maternal will to live were intensified with an HIV+ child.
29. Mothers of HIV+ children were ambivalent about revealing their HIV to them, suppressing or isolating them from the diagnosis and psychoimmunizing them against its treatment.
30. Mothers of HIV+ children selectively used medical treatment in efforts to normalize their lives and to protect them from the physical and emotional harms of HIV and its treatment.
31. Mothers addressed uncertainty over the HIV+ child's sense of the future by integrating future-oriented thinking into present-oriented actions, and having short-term goals that can be stretched to longer-term goals.
32. Mothers addressed uncertainty over the management of the HIV+ child by overprotection, over-reaction, filtering information, seeking information from multiple sources, managing the child's environment, and using outside agencies.

Vertical & horizontal transmission to fetus and children
33. Women had varying knowledge, concerns, and interpretations of, and used various strategies to address, the risk of HIV transmission to fetuses and children.
34. Mothers felt guilt/remorse/blame (from children or others) over their perceived deficits as mothers, and for infecting children.

AZT/ARV use in pregnancy

35. Barriers to the use of AZT in pregnancy, whether or not women were willing to use it, included: fear of toxicity to the baby, side effects, and drug resistance; belief that it was unnecessary if the mother was healthy; having given birth to a healthy child without AZT; and fear of stigma for children.

36. Facilitators of intention to use AZT in pregnancy, whether or not women intended to use it, included: belief in its efficacy and that they owed it to the baby; the influence of or good relations with MDs; others having had healthy babies with AZT; having given birth to a healthy child with AZT; and fear of losing services or health care if they were not taking ARVs while pregnant.

Medical & self care

37. Mothers identified self-care as important to being able to live as long as possible to take care of their children, but child care took precedence over maternal self-care.

38. Non-HIV–related factors, including child care, facilitated or impeded utilization of health and social services.

39. Mothers avoided HIV clinics and infectious disease specialists for fear of having their HIV status exposed.

40. Fear of HIV transmission to child was both a motivating factor and a barrier to utilizing prenatal care services.

41. A barrier to seeking prenatal care was fear of breaches in confidentiality, providers' fears of HIV, and exposure to sicker patients.

42. Mothers sought information for comfort and to make decisions.

Custody, legacy, and the future

43. Mothers had concerns over child care and/or placement, especially as maternal disease worsened and/or after maternal death.

44. Often viewing custody planning as a symbol for giving up and accepting death, mothers exhibited no plan or a reluctance to have completed legal documentation concerning custody, but identified individuals to assume custody, primarily their mothers.

45. Mothers wanted to leave a positive legacy, including sharing with their children advice, family secrets, values, and special memories and mementos.

46. Mothers hoped to prolong their lives in order to accomplish motherhood goals, but felt time was running out as they viewed HIV as a death sentence.

47. Mothers felt hope and hopelessness for the future.

48. The differences among women in planning were related to the length of time since diagnosis and symptoms.

49. Voluntary or enforced separation from children was more difficult to deal with than HIV itself.

50. Mothers engaged in anticipatory separation to prepare their children for emotional independence after maternal death.

51. Mothers concentrated on the present rather than the future.

Reproductive decision making

52. Both HIV-related and unrelated factors were involved in women's decisions to conceive, continue, or terminate pregnancies, with the same or different moralities, desires, risk assessments, or circumstances leading to the same or different decisions.

53. Women were hurt or angered by providers who offered misinformation, conveyed that they ought not to reproduce, conveyed advice in a hurtful way, or tried to coerce them concerning reproduction.
54. Women perceived having HIV as the loss of the opportunity to have children.
55. Women generally made reproductive decisions alone, but believed reproductive decisions ought to be a woman's alone.
56. Women wanted more information, or reported a lack of information on which to base reproductive decisions.
57. Women framed reproductive decisions in religious terms.
58. Both absolute & contextual moral reasoning (justice vs. care) drove reproductive decision making.
59. Women had strong desires to have children despite concerns about perinatal transmission.
60. Women's mothers were most important to them in making reproductive decisions.
61. Women had strong feelings that women who used drugs should not have children.
62. Women's justifications for wanting a baby included: offering reasons for why a child would not be HIV+, or why they would be better mothers; other infected women having had healthy babies; the belief that AZT can help women have healthy babies; faith in God; being healthy and young; and being better able to raise a child now.

Conceptual syntheses
63. *Defensive motherhood:* Faced with a double bind, by which women are supposed to want motherhood and become mothers, but not if they are HIV+, mothers engaged in defensive mothering, which involved strategies to prevent the spread of HIV and stigma, prepare children for a motherless future, and maintain a positive attitude.
64. *Eternal motherhood:* Eternal aspects of motherhood were characterized by anticipating future events, giving advice for life, and promising to be eternally available in spirit, even after physical death.
65. *Redefined motherhood:* To retain the maternal role in the face of threats to motherhood, mothers redefined motherhood, emphasizing tasks that could be maintained despite changing health status and, when those tasks could no longer be performed, reframing the role of mother as one of oversight of children's well-being.
66. *Protective motherhood:* "La Protectora" is an intensification of the mother role following diagnosis of HIV infection, in which women bargain for the life and health of their children.
67. *Redefining treatment:* A form of protective motherhood whereby the desire to compensate for transmitting HIV and societal views of motherhood and HIV led women to protect HIV+ children by continually redefining the nature and boundaries of treatment of the child.

TABLE 6.1 Edited Findings Pertaining to Motherhood From Four Studies of HIV-Positive Women

Report and purpose	Edited findings
Andrews, 1993 Motherhood	Children are important sources of social support, even when not in maternal custody.
	Mothers have strong physical and psychological attachments to their children.
	Mothers universally struggle with whether to disclose their HIV diagnosis to young children.
	Most mothers have decided against disclosure to children.
	A reason for not disclosing is the perceived inability of young children to understand or deal with impending maternal death.
	The decision not to disclose to children means that mothers will not have to spend time and energy soothing their worries.
	The results of decisions about disclosure have ramifications.
	Disclosure to a young child may lead to unwanted disclosure to neighbors, friends, and acquaintances.
	Mothers worry about how a seropositive child will be treated by others.
	The burden of secrecy is heavy when both mother and child are HIV+.
	Keeping the secret of HIV is complicated.
	Mothers worry that their own physical condition will make it impossible to avoid disclosure to their children.
	Mothers wonder if it might be preferable to discontinue contact with children before their condition becomes difficult for the child to bear.
	HIV+ mothers, like other mothers, perceive both supportive and burdensome aspects in their relationship with their children.
	Children are supportive by their mere presence and thereby decrease feelings of isolation associated with HIV.
	Children are supportive by offering affection and unconditional love.
	Children are supportive by preserving mothers' attachment to the world.
	Children's support buffers effects of HIV-related stigmatization.
	Children are supportive by forcing mothers to approach life positively, not to give in or give up.

(continued)

TABLE 6.1 Edited Findings Pertaining to Motherhood From Four Studies of HIV-Positive Women *(Continued)*

Report and purpose	Edited findings
Andrews *(cont'd)* Motherhood	Child care and the mother-child bond are a source of maternal self-esteem.
	Because children are vulnerable and needy, they distract mothers from their own vulnerability.
	Children are supportive by their ability to prevent mothers from engaging in high risk behaviors, especially drug use.
	Motherhood is burdensome because of concerns about the eventual placement of surviving children, especially a seropositive child.
	Motherhood is burdensome because of fears for seropositive child's health, hospitalizations, and eventual death.
	Mothers of seropositive children spend much time and energy caring for them, which detracts from their own health.
	Children are burdensome because they reduce maternal privacy as mother is usually sole caregiver and never alone.
	Obtaining child care is a problem for seropositive mothers, especially when the child is also seropositive.
	Children are burdensome when they react angrily to their mother's HIV.
Armstrong, 1996 Motherhood	(In the context of uncertainty) Mothers were uncertain about the course of HIV disease in their children.
	Mothers were uncertain about the management of their HIV+ child's health, including appraisal, medical treatment, and home care.
	Mothers were uncertain about the HIV+ child having a sense of its own future.
	Mothers were uncertain about disclosing HIV to children.
	Mothers were concerned about the ability of children to understand the physiological and psychological implications of having HIV.
	Mothers were concerned about the ability of children to keep HIV secret.
	Mothers were concerned about children's reaction to disclosure.
	Mothers were concerned about children's reaction to them after disclosure.

TABLE 6.1 *(Continued)*

Report and purpose	Edited findings
	Mothers expressed concerns that their HIV+ children would not have a sense of their own future.
	Mothers were uncertain whether they or child would die first.
	Maternal strategies used to combat uncertainty over management of child's HIV included overprotection, over-reaction, filtering information, seeking information from multiple sources, managing the child's environment, and using outside agencies.
	Maternal strategies used to combat uncertainty over disclosure of HIV to child included not telling, timing the disclosure, selective disclosure.
	Maternal strategies used to combat uncertainty over child sense of the future included integrating future-oriented thinking into present-oriented actions, having short-term goals that can be stretched to longer-term goals.
	Maternal strategies used to combat uncertainty over maternal or child death included arranging legal custody, seeking support before and after child's death.
	(In the context of HIV stigma)
	All mothers reported stigmatization attributed to HIV infection.
	Mothers reported being stigmatized by people close and distant to them.
	Mothers reported overt and covert stigmatization.
	Mothers experienced triple stigma associated with fear of lethal contagion, association between HIV and drug abuse, and promiscuity, and with maternal transmission to "innocent" child.
	Mothers managed stigma by not disclosing and passing.
	(In context of finding out that they have HIV)
	Maternal HIV is often diagnosed during pregnancy or after the child's diagnosis.
	This timing of diagnosis forces women to face death at a time generally associated with life.
	The timing of diagnosis (before or during, or concurrent with their child's diagnosis) entails different kinds of experiences and decisions.
	All mothers, whether diagnosed independently or concurrently with their children's diagnoses, indicated their belief that they would neither have children nor become pregnant in the future.

(continued)

TABLE 6.1 Edited Findings Pertaining to Motherhood From Four Studies of HIV-Positive Women *(Continued)*

Report and purpose	Edited findings
Armstrong *(cont'd)* Motherhood	Even mothers who had knowledge of the reduced perinatal transmission rate with ARV therapy during pregnancy believed they would not risk pregnancy.
	All pregnant women in their third month of pregnancy faced the decision of whether to continue their pregnancy.
	Factors influencing pregnant women's decision include stage of pregnancy, pressure from medical staff, and religious or moral beliefs.
	When asked whether they would consider abortion if the stage of their pregnancies did not preclude abortion as an option, seven mothers would not have considered abortion and two were not sure. Eleven reported that they would, or probably would have, terminated their pregnancy. (Eight mothers were diagnosed during their pregnancy. Two mothers knew of their diagnosis prior to becoming pregnant. Ten mothers were diagnosed after their child had been diagnosed with HIV.)
	Mothers faced the dilemma of whether to treat their children and/or themselves, and which treatment to choose.
	Mothers reported their decisions to receive treatment (AZT) were strongly influenced by their physician's advice.
	Mothers' decisions not to receive treatment were primarily attributed to fears surrounding current drug therapies.
	Mothers' reactions to diagnosis, especially depression, initially interfered with their ability to care for child.
	Having an HIV+ child was a primary motivator to enter, continue, and/or return to drug recovery programs.
	(In context of effect on family)
	All the mothers expressed sadness at some aspect of their maternal role.
	All mothers expressed the difficulty in establishing or maintaining their role as mother at some period during their HIV illness.
	Mothers of only children discussed their difficulty in establishing an identity because they believed the likelihood of mother or child surviving together was extremely poor. (Fifteen children were the only children in the family. One-fourth of their mothers were 39 to 41 years old at the time of diagnosis.)
	Mothers, 20 to 35 years old at the time of diagnosis, struggled with accepting their role of "mother with a dying child" and the loss of their identity as a mother.

TABLE 6.1 *(Continued)*

Report and purpose	Edited findings

Mothers with other children struggled more to maintain their maternal identity, wanted to keep things as normal as possible, until their health or their child's health required them to alter their family routine.

Mothers with other children wanted to maintain their identity as mother, rather than as person with AIDS, and reported denying or suppressing their diagnosis.

Several mothers wanted to preserve their identity as mother after maternal death.

More than half of mothers described their relationship with their children as special because of the bond formed by their dual HIV infection.

Mothers who were asymptomatic were more likely to stress qualities of the mother-child relationship as supportive, providing affection, and giving the mother a reason to live.

Mothers with HIV-related symptoms or whose child was symptomatic emphasized the caregiving aspects of the relationship, reporting the need for respite but also hesitant to leave their child.

(In the context of blame)

The mothers reported feelings of being blamed by others and blaming themselves for their child's HIV infection.

Mothers who reported feeling blamed by others referred to both covert and overt behaviors by the medical care providers, HIV– partners, or family members.

Nearly one-fourth of the mothers felt that it was likely that they might have to face being blamed by their own children in the future.

HIV+ mothers were also blamed by other HIV+ mothers, although less directly. Within the group of HIV+ mothers, mothers referred to other mothers by their mode of transmission in derogatory terms (e.g., "dirty" or drug-abusing mothers get help that "clean" mothers do not).

Nearly three-fourths of the mothers blamed themselves for having been the vector for their child's HIV infection because they used injection drugs, did not take birth control precautions, or maintained a relationship with an HIV+ partner.

One-fourth of the mothers reported they would probably blame themselves if the child's condition worsened or the child died if they did not accept current drug treatment.

(continued)

TABLE 6.1 Edited Findings Pertaining to Motherhood From Four Studies of HIV-Positive Women *(Continued)*

Report and purpose	Edited findings
Armstrong *(cont'd)* Motherhood	Mothers cited reasons for not taking drugs, including the experimental nature of drug therapies, their uncertain efficacy or long-term outcomes, and the child's current good health state.
	Several mothers acknowledged that they would probably blame themselves if their child died or became worse, if they were to leave the child during respite care.
	Feelings of anger and hate were expressed toward partners who reportedly knew but did not disclose their HIV, whom they blame for infecting them and their child.
	(In context of feeling helpless)
	Mothers described feeling helpless to help their child when the child suffered an HIV-related illness, the illness became acute, or treatment decisions for clinical trials or drug therapies were recommended.
	Nearly half of mothers felt helpless because they were unable to provide their HIV+ child with anticipatory preparation for their illness course due to the unpredictability and variability of the disease course.
	One-fourth of mothers felt helpless to offer their child hope during chronic or acute phases of their illness.
	Mothers felt helpless when facing treatment decisions for self and child, primarily feeling unqualified to select the initial treatment(s), much less challenge ongoing therapies.
	Some mothers felt helpless to change the course of the disease for their children or themselves or to even manage the symptoms of the infection.
	Nearly all mothers felt helpless in finding emotional support specific to the needs of being an HIV+ mother with an HIV+ child due to the non-existence of community-based HIV+ mother/HIV+ child support groups.
	Mothers identified the need to provide emotional support to the siblings of the HIV+ child, including providing reassurance or anticipatory preparation to the siblings during acute stages of illness, and disclosing the diagnosis.
	Mothers felt helpless to offer the siblings reassurance about a positive outcome for their HIV+ brother or sister due to the unpredictability of HIV infection.
	(In the context of hope)
	Nearly half the mothers described feeling hopeless about their dual HIV infection.

TABLE 6.1 *(Continued)*

Report and purpose	Edited findings
	Over half of mothers felt hopeful.
	Six mothers reported hope and hopelessness.
	Nearly one-third of mothers were hopeful they would cure the child with or without treatment or child would grow out of it.
	One-half of women hoped for treatments to slow the virus or decrease opportunistic infections.
	Hopelessness was generally grounded in mothers' sense of the fatality of HIV infection.
	One-fourth of mothers attributed fatalism to their interactions with their therapists or physicians.
	(In the context of disclosure)
	Mothers were continually faced with the decision of whether to disclose their own or their children's HIV infection to others and even to their own children.
	Mothers based their decision to tell their HIV+ child and/or the siblings on what they perceived the child would be able to understand about both the physiological and psychosocial implications of HIV infection.
	Nearly all mothers believed they would tell their child and/or their siblings when they reached a certain level of understanding, which they associated with the tenth birthday.
	When they perceived that exposure of the infection might result in their HIV+ child and/or their other children (who did not know diagnosis) finding out, they did not disclose.
	In deciding to tell, mothers considered the other party's need to know, including health or school.
	The need to know focused on the risk of transmission to others and the medical needs of the child or themselves.
	(In context of coping)
	Maintaining health was the primary strategy for coping to prolong survival to benefit from medical advances in HIV treatments.
	Mothers sought support from family, friends, and AIDS agencies to obtain respite from the emotional stressors of being the sole care provider.
	Mothers sought support from other HIV+ mothers with HIV+ children seeking reassurance, empathy or comfort, and sharing information.
	Mothers sought to increase their knowledge to select or deny treatment for themselves or their child.

(continued)

TABLE 6.1 Edited Findings Pertaining to Motherhood From Four Studies of HIV-Positive Women (Continued)

Report and purpose	Edited findings
Armstrong (cont'd) Motherhood	Seeking information also served to decrease mothers' feelings of anxiety related to the uncertainty of the trajectory of HIV infection and/or AIDS.
	Mothers focused on obtaining information about current and upcoming clinical trials, treatments, and clinical markers.
	Primary sources of information were HIV/AIDS centers, educational programs, and their primary-care health care providers.
Black, 2002 Disclosure	Deciding not to disclose to the larger community was sometimes done to protect the children from courtesy stigma.
	Revealing their HIV diagnoses to the larger community raised the possibility that the children might be stigmatized.
	Most women had elected not to disclose their diagnosis to their children.
	Typically, the children were deemed "too young" to understand the implications of the virus or there was a concern the child might inadvertently reveal the diagnosis to others.
	Timing was an important issue when calculating when to disclose their HIV diagnosis to their children. Many women discussed their plans to tell their children when they were older and presumably more able to understand the illness and its ramifications.
	As with the other women, even full disclosers did not tell their children because they were considered too young to understand the implications of the diagnosis.
Ciambrone, 2001 HIV compared to other traumas	Being separated from their children was among the events deemed more destructive than HIV.
	Many of the women had to give up custody of their children, either voluntarily or involuntarily.
	Seven women with children under 18 were noncustodial mothers, whereas nine women had custody of their children.
	Two women had custody of their children, but had been temporarily separated from their children in the past.
	For some women, mother-child separation was a deliberate decision to secure the best care.
	Other women were forcibly separated from their children, mostly because of substance abuse.

TABLE 6.1 *(Continued)*

Report and purpose	Edited findings
	Women who experienced separation from children as a severely disruptive event were forced to relinquish a role that gave a sense of purpose and continuity to their lives.
	Illness was easier to incorporate into women's biographies than separation from children.
	Women found that dealing with the feelings of failure and guilt that resulted from losing their children transcended the challenges associated with HIV.
	Some women desperately wanted to become mothers but did not see pregnancy as an option, given the risk of vertical transmission.
	HIV made motherhood an elusive goal.

TABLE 6.2 Example of Grouping: Positive Features of Motherhood

Study	Edited findings
Andrews, 1993	Children are important sources of social support, even when not in maternal custody.
	Mothers have strong physical and psychological attachments to their children.
	Mothers universally struggle with whether to disclose their HIV diagnosis to young children.
	Most mothers have decided against disclosure to children.
	A reason for not disclosing is the perceived inability of young children to understand or deal with impending maternal death.
	The decision not to disclose to children means that mothers will not have to spend time and energy soothing their worries.
	The results of decisions about disclosure have ramifications.
	Disclosure to a young child may lead to unwanted disclosure to neighbors, friends, and acquaintances.
	Mothers worry about how a seropositive child will be treated by others.
	The burden of secrecy is heavy when both mother and child are HIV+.
	Keeping the secret of HIV is complicated.
	Mothers worry that their own physical condition will make it impossible to avoid disclosure to their children.
	Mothers wonder if it might be preferable to discontinue contact with children before their condition becomes difficult for the child to bear.
	HIV+ mothers, like other mothers, perceive both supportive and burdensome aspects in their relationship with their children.
	Children are supportive by their mere presence and thereby decrease feelings of isolation associated with HIV.
	Children are supportive by offering affection and unconditional love.
	Children are supportive by preserving mothers' attachment to the world.
	Children's support buffers effects of HIV-related stigmatization.
	Children are supportive by forcing mothers to approach life positively, not to give in or give up.
	Child care and the mother-child bond are a source of maternal self-esteem.
	Because children are vulnerable and needy, they distract mothers from their own vulnerability.

TABLE 6.2 *(Continued)*

Study	Edited findings
	Children are supportive by their ability to prevent mothers from engaging in high risk behaviors, especially drug use.
	Motherhood is burdensome because of concerns about the eventual placement of surviving children, especially a seropositive child.
	Motherhood is burdensome because of fears for seropositive child's health, hospitalizations, and eventual death.
	Mothers of seropositive children spend much time and energy caring for them, which detracts from their own health.
	Children are burdensome because they reduce maternal privacy as mother is usually sole caregiver and never alone.
	Obtaining child care is a problem for seropositive mothers, especially when the child is also seropositive.
	Children are burdensome when they react angrily to their mother's HIV.
Bunting, 1999	A factor promoting medical and self-care was staying healthy for children.
	Many women spoke of their children as the focus of their lives, and as a reason for living.
	A factor impeding medical and self-care was obtaining child care.
	Even with limited resources, women always chose to take care of their children first.
Ciambrone, 2002	For women with children, disclosing was perhaps the hardest thing they have ever had to do.
	Some of the women noted the difficulties of being a mother with HIV infection.
	Many women noted the strength they derive from mothering, which in turn helped them create or maintain a sense of normalcy.
	Women who did not have intravenous drug use histories were more likely to highlight their children's role in their repair process than those with intravenous drug use histories.
	Of the women who noted that caring for their children helped them cope with their illness, 59% had been living with HIV infection for 7 or more years, and 41% had the virus for less than 7 years.
	Mothers often referred to their children as great sources of motivation.
	Although most women talked about how their children provided emotional support, relatively few reported that they provided instrumental assistance.

(continued)

TABLE 6.2 Example of Grouping: Positive Features of Motherhood *(Continued)*

Study	Edited findings
	Children generally took their mothers' news fairly well and offered support, often just by being loving.
	Several women (n = 9), however, reported that one or more of their children were unsympathetic, seemingly uninterested, or outright cruel when they informed them of their serostatus.
	Children's reactions early on proved to be a good indicator of eventual support patterns.
	Some mothers continued to provide emotional and practical support to their children but received little succor in return.
	With the exception of one woman, all women with children over the age of 13 had disclosed their illness. Women with children < 13 reported that they planned to tell their children, but felt that they were too young to carry such a heavy burden and/or understand what it means to have HIV.
Ingram, 2000	(Most women were already mothers. Nine women had decided to continue their pregnancies when diagnosed as HIV+. Three women knew of their HIV before choosing to become pregnant. Three women were actively struggling with whether to become pregnant.)
	HIV+ women face a double bind, by which women are supposed to want motherhood and become mothers, but not if they are HIV+.
	Many women believed that health care providers saw reproduction as bad because of their HIV infection.
	Women embraced the idea of giving birth and were hurt and angered by negative social messages condemning reproduction in HIV+ women.
	Women feared and worried about perinatal transmission to fetus.
	For three mothers with HIV+ babies, these babies were the reason they decided not to have more children.
	By choosing to have more children, women also feared transmitting HIV to their partners.
	Women struggled with the social ambivalence directed at them as mothers.
	HIV made it hard for women to fulfill the social expectations of mothering.
	Women had many caretaking responsibilities.
	Women felt unable to mother effectively because of the physical demands of HIV.
	Fatigue was a common problem for mothers.
	Mothers embraced mothering and articulated the importance of their children in their lives.

TABLE 6.2 *(Continued)*

Study	Edited findings
	Mothers identified their children as a reasons for being, continuing to fight to survive and to stay healthy.
	In condition of stigma, mothers gave to and received from children unconditional love.
	Mothers feared they had a negative impact on the health and well-being of their children.
	Mothers felt a sense of temporal urgency related to their children.
	Children of HIV+ mothers became hypervigilant guardian children, caring for the physical and emotional needs of their mothers and essentially assuming the role of mother.
	Mothers were concerned about the negative effects on their children's mental health of assuming adult roles.
	Mothers struggled with whether to tell their children about their HIV.
	Eight of the 18 mothers had disclosed their HIV status to their children.
	Mothers understood the importance of disclosure in helping prepare their children for the future.
	Mothers attempted to protect children by not telling them about their HIV.
	Mothers who chose not to tell their children described feeling constant anxiety that their children would hear the news in a cruel manner from strangers.
	Another major concern about disclosing to the children was the possibility of the children repeating the family secret to others.
	Mothers grappled with how to tell their children not to tell others without conveying a sense of wrongdoing.
	Mothers were aware that children sensed something wrong.
	Confidentiality and anonymity were of highest importance because of the threat to mothers and children posed by the stigma of HIV.
Valdez, 1999	(La Protectora)
	The majority of women discovered their positive status during pregnancy.
	Most women were pregnant at diagnosis or chose to get pregnant knowing their positive status.
	The pregnancy and ultimately the child became the impetus that appeared to take the women to "Ofrecer."
	Ofrecer is "an offer to change," and is characterized by a woman's negotiating with God on behalf of her child.

(continued)

TABLE 6.2 Example of Grouping: Positive Features of Motherhood *(Continued)*

Study	Edited findings
	The Hispanic woman during the Ofrecer stage promises to do good, namely live for her child and reveal her status to benefit others. Her exchange is not for herself or for more time but for the life of her child.
	Most of the women had not told their children of their HIV.
	Despite lack of disclosure to children, most women had made arrangements for their children after their death.
	Most women left significant family members with detailed instructions on the disposition of the children. Other women wrote lengthy letters to each of their children, to be given to them upon their death.
	Other women hoped that they would live long enough to let their children grow to more of an acceptable age to tolerate the news.
	Some of the women expressed more fear of disclosure for their children and families.
	Day-to-day, women cared for families while struggling with their own physical and emotional well-being.
	Women's strength to live came partly from being mothers.
	Women saw their lives as important because they had to care for their children and their families.
	When faced with death, women chose the path of living for their child rather than accepting to die.
	Their decision to live and emerge as La Protectora was influenced by the birth of their child and the revelation of the child's negative status.

Note. Groupings are **bolded.**

TABLE 6.3 Findings Pertaining to Motherhood With Frequency Effect Sizes = > 20%

Abstracted findings (N=67)	Published reports (N=36)	Unpublished reports (N=20)	Frequency effect sizes
14. Mothers struggled with whether to disclose their HIV to their children, worried about the effects of disclosure on child and maternal welfare and the maternal-child relationship, and engaged in strategies to disclose or to delay or avoid disclosing their HIV status to their children.	Andrews Barnes Black Ciambrone (networks) **Faithfull** Goggin Hackl **Ingram (double)** **Ingram (stigma)** Marcenko Moneyham Regan-Kubinski Santacroce Schrimshaw, Siegel Semple Smith **Valdez** Walker Winstead	Armstrong Arnold Bennett Caba **Ciambrone** **Faithfull** Gosling Hendrixson **Ingram** Loriz-Lim Palyo Ross Tangenberg	57%
43. Mothers had concerns over child care and/or placement, especially as maternal disease worsened and/or after maternal death.	Andrews **Faithfull** Goggin	**Valdez** Wright Armstrong Bonifas Caba Ciambrone **Faithfull** Frey	44%

(continued)

TABLE 6.3 Findings Pertaining to Motherhood With Frequency Effect Sizes = > 20% (Continued)

Abstracted findings (N=67)	Published reports (N=36)	Unpublished reports (N=20)	Frequency effect sizes
	Hackl	Gosling	
		Hendrixson	
	Ingram (defensive)	**Ingram**	
	Litwak	Loriz-Lim	
	Marcenko	Palyo	
	Regan-Kubinski		
	Semple		
	Valdez	**Valdez**	
	Van Loon	**Van Loon**	
	Walker	Wright	
	Winstead		
1. Children were the main reasons to live, fight, get off drugs, care for oneself, and avoid risky behaviors.	Andrews	Armstrong	40%
	Bunting	Bennett	
		Bonifas	
		Caba	
		Cameron	
	Ciambrone (networks)	**Ciambrone**	
		Faithfull	
		Gosling	
	Ingram (defensive)	**Ingram**	
	Ingram (double)		
	Goggin	Loriz-Lim	
	Hutchison		
	Kass		
	Regan-Kubinski		
	Sankar		

This landscape table is printed rotated on the page. Columns: Finding | Reports | Reports | Effect size.

Finding	Reports	Reports	Effect size
2. Whether their children were in or out of their care or custody, being a mother was central to women's lives: a source of self-esteem, strength, normalcy, inspiration, pride, hope, joy, sense of well-being, & sense of self as a whole woman.	**Valdez** **Van Loon** Walker Wesley	**Valdez** **Van Loon**	26%
33. Women had varying knowledge, concerns, and interpretations of, and used various strategies to address, the risk of HIV transmission to fetuses and children.	Andrews **Ciambrone (networks)** Goggin Hutchison Kass Sowell **Valdez** **Van Loon** Walker Wesley **Faithfull** Hackl **Ingram (double)** Napravnik Semple Smith Sowell Walker	Caba **Ciambrone** Faithfull Loriz-Lim Tangenberg **Valdez** **Van Loon** Bonifas Ciambrone **Faithfull** Frey **Ingram** Tangenberg	22%
8. Mothers worried about the negative impact of maternal HIV (the illness itself and/or its stigma) on their children, including their negative reactions to it and others' negative reactions to their children.	Andrews Barnes **Ciambrone (networks)** Hackl	Armstrong **Ciambrone**	21%

(continued)

TABLE 6.3 Findings Pertaining to Motherhood With Frequency Effect Sizes = > 20% *(Continued)*

Abstracted findings (N=67)	Published reports (N=36)	Unpublished reports (N=20)	Frequency effect sizes
	Ingram (double) **Ingram (stigma)** Marcenko Santacroce Semple **Van Loon** Walker	**Ingram** **Van Loon**	
52. Both HIV-related and unrelated factors were involved in women's decisions to conceive, continue, or terminate pregnancies, with the same or different moralities, desires, risk assessments, or circumstances leading to the same or different decisions.	Hutchison **Ingram (double)** Kass Siegel, Schrimshaw Sowell Walker Wesley	Armstrong Bonifas Faithfull Frey **Ingram**	20%

Note. Related reports are **bolded** and aligned.

TABLE 6.4 Four Studies With Largest Intensity Effect Sizes of Findings Pertaining to Motherhood

Author	Findings	Effect sizes
Faithfull, 1992 (thesis)	1. Children were the main reasons to live, fight, get off drugs, care for oneself, and avoid risky behaviors.	34%
	2. Whether their children were in or out of their care or custody, being a mother was central to women's lives: a source of self-esteem, strength, normalcy, inspiration, pride, hope, joy, sense of well-being, & sense of self as a whole woman.	
	4. HIV had a positive impact on mothering, especially in drug-abusing women and women living with HIV for a longer time.	
	5. Mothers reported strong physical and psychological attachments to their children, and intensification of the maternal role.	
	7. Mothers viewed children as their legacy, final acts of creation, rescuers, saviors, and fulfillers of their unfulfilled dreams.	
	9. The combination of motherhood and HIV was physically demanding.	
	10. Maternity/life was often the context for HIV diagnosis/death in women.	
	11. Often the sole caregivers, mothers reported concerns, frustrations, and difficulties disciplining children.	
	12. Mothers, especially those who had abused drugs or were ill, struggled to establish, maintain, and/or preserve maternal identity while children were out of their care, during illness, and after maternal death.	
	14. Mothers struggled with whether to disclose their HIV to their children, worried about the effects of disclosure on child and maternal welfare and the maternal-child relationship, and engaged in strategies to disclose or to delay or avoid disclosing their HIV status to their children.	
	24. Mothers had special concerns about, hopes for, and were consumed with the health, illness care, future, and placement of HIV+ children.	

(continued)

TABLE 6.4 Four Studies With Largest Intensity Effect Sizes of Findings Pertaining to Motherhood *(Continued)*

Author	Findings	Effect sizes
	25. Mothers reported instances, or worried about the negative effects, of HIV– child role reversal, or had adult expectations of their assuming a mother or caretaking role.	
	33. Women had varying knowledge, concerns, and interpretations of, and used various strategies to address, the risk of HIV transmission to fetuses and children.	
	34. Mothers felt guilt/remorse/blame (from children or others) over their perceived deficits as mothers, and for infecting children.	
	43. Mothers had concerns over child care and/or placement, especially as maternal disease worsened and/or after maternal death.	
	44. Often viewing custody planning as a symbol for giving up and accepting death, mothers exhibited no plan or a reluctance to have completed legal documentation concerning custody, but identified individuals to assume custody, primarily their mothers.	
	45. Mothers wanted to leave a positive legacy, including sharing with their children advice, family secrets, values, and special memories and mementos.	
	47. Mothers felt hope and hopelessness for the future.	
	48. The differences among women in planning were related to the length of time since diagnosis and symptoms.	
	52. Both HIV-related and unrelated factors were involved in women's decisions to conceive, continue, or terminate pregnancies, with the same or different moralities, desires, risk assessments, or circumstances leading to the same or different decisions.	
	53. Women were hurt or angered by providers who offered misinformation, conveyed that they ought not to reproduce, conveyed advice in a hurtful way, or tried to coerce them concerning reproduction.	

31%

55. Women generally made reproductive decisions alone, but believed reproductive decisions ought to be a woman's alone.

58. Both absolute & contextual moral reasoning (justice vs. care) drove reproductive decision making.

Ingram, 1996 (dissertation)

1. Children were the main reasons to live, fight, get off drugs, care for oneself, and avoid risky behaviors.

3. Children were important sources of physical, practical, emotional, and social support, and unconditional love to their mothers, buffering the negative effects of HIV.

8. Mothers worried about the negative impact of maternal HIV (the illness itself and/or its stigma) on their children, including their negative reactions to it and others' negative reactions to their children.

9. The combination of motherhood and HIV was physically demanding.

14. Mothers struggled with whether to disclose their HIV to their children, worried about the effects of disclosure on child and maternal welfare and the maternal-child relationship, and engaged in strategies to disclose or to delay or avoid disclosing their HIV status to their children.

15. Women with children were subject to the triple stigmatization (of drug abuse, promiscuity, and infecting the innocent), and reported stigmatization attributed to HIV infection.

21. By telling others about their HIV, mothers garnered support for themselves and their children, protected others from HIV, but risked more disclosure, rejection, and exposing loved ones to pain.

22. By not telling others, mothers protected themselves and their children from the threat of disclosure, but cut themselves and their children off from sources of support, and left their families and friends unprepared to deal with their impending death.

(continued)

TABLE 6.4 Four Studies With Largest Intensity Effect Sizes of Findings Pertaining to Motherhood (*Continued*)

Author	Findings	Effect sizes
	23. Mothers wanted and acted to protect all their children.	
	24. Mothers had special concerns about, hopes for, and were consumed with the health, illness care, future, and placement of HIV+ children.	
	25. Mothers reported instances, or worried about the negative effects, of HIV– child role reversal, or had adult expectations of their assuming a mother or caretaking role.	
	33. Women had varying knowledge, concerns, and interpretations of, and used various strategies to address, the risk of HIV transmission to fetuses and children.	
	37. Mothers identified self-care as important to being able to live as long as possible to take care of their children, but child care took precedence over maternal self-care.	
	39. Mothers avoided HIV clinics and infectious disease specialists for fear of having their HIV status exposed.	
	43. Mothers had concerns over child care and/or placement, especially as maternal disease worsened and/or after maternal death.	
	44. Often viewing custody planning as a symbol for giving up and accepting death, mothers exhibited no plan or a reluctance to have completed legal documentation concerning custody, but identified individuals to assume custody, primarily their mothers.	
	45. Mothers wanted to leave a positive legacy, including sharing with their children advice, family secrets, values, and special memories and mementos.	
	46. Mothers hoped to prolong their lives in order to accomplish motherhood goals, but felt time was running out as they viewed HIV as a death sentence.	
	52. Both HIV-related and unrelated factors were involved in women's decisions to conceive, continue, or terminate pregnancies, with the same or different moralities, desires, risk assessments, or circumstances leading to the same or different decisions.	

53. Women were hurt or angered by providers who offered misinformation, conveyed that they ought not to reproduce, conveyed advice in a hurtful way, or tried to coerce them concerning reproduction.

56. Women wanted more information, or reported a lack of information on which to base reproductive decisions.

Armstrong, 1996   30%
(dissertation)

1. Children were the main reasons to live, fight, get off drugs, care for oneself, and avoid risky behaviors.

8. Mothers worried about the negative impact of maternal HIV (the illness itself and/or its stigma) on their children, including their negative reactions to it and others' negative reactions to their children.

9. The combination of motherhood and HIV was physically demanding.

10. Maternity/life was often the context for HIV diagnosis/death in women.

12. Mothers, especially those who had abused drugs or were ill, struggled to establish, maintain, and/or preserve maternal identity while children were out of their care, during illness, and after maternal death.

14. Mothers struggled with whether to disclose their HIV to their children, worried about the effects of disclosure on child and maternal welfare and the maternal-child relationship, and engaged in strategies to disclose or to delay or avoid disclosing their HIV status to their children.

15. Women with children were subject to the triple stigmatization (of drug abuse, promiscuity, and infecting the innocent), and reported stigmatization attributed to HIV infection.

24. Mothers had special concerns about, hopes for, and were consumed with the health, illness care, future, and placement of HIV+ children.

26. Mother-child relations changed with the progress of maternal or child HIV disease.

28. Maternal attention and attachment, mother-child relations, and maternal will to live were intensified with an HIV+ child.

(continued)

TABLE 6.4 Four Studies With Largest Intensity Effect Sizes of Findings Pertaining to Motherhood *(Continued)*

Author	Findings	Effect sizes
	31. Mothers addressed uncertainty over the HIV+ child's sense of the future by integrating future-oriented thinking into present-oriented actions, and having short-term goals that can be stretched to longer-term goals.	
	32. Mothers addressed uncertainty over the management of the HIV+ child by overprotection, over-reaction, filtering information, seeking information from multiple sources, managing the child's environment, and using outside agencies.	
	34. Mothers felt guilt/remorse/blame (from children or others) over their perceived deficits as mothers, and for infecting children.	
	35. Barriers to the use of AZT in pregnancy, whether or not women were willing to use it, included: fear of toxicity to the baby, side effects, and drug resistance; belief that it was unnecessary if the mother was healthy; having given birth to a healthy child without AZT; and fear of stigma for children.	
	36. Facilitators of intention to use AZT in pregnancy, whether or not women intended to use it, included: belief in its efficacy and that they owed it to the baby, the influence of or good relations with MDs, others having had healthy babies with AZT, having given birth to a healthy child with AZT, and fear of losing services or health care if they were not taking ARVs while pregnant.	
	37. Mothers identified self-care as important to being able to live as long as possible to take care of their children, but child care took precedence over maternal self-care.	
	42. Mothers sought information for comfort and to make decisions.	
	43. Mothers had concerns over child care and/or placement, especially as maternal disease worsened and/or after maternal death.	
	47. Mothers felt hope and hopelessness for the future.	

Walker, 1996, 1998
(dissertation, book)

25%

52. Both HIV-related and unrelated factors were involved in women's decisions to conceive, continue, or terminate pregnancies, with the same or different moralities, desires, risk assessments, or circumstances leading to the same or different decisions.

1. Children were the main reasons to live, fight, get off drugs, care for oneself, and avoid risky behaviors.

2. Whether their children were in or out of their care or custody, being a mother was central to women's lives: a source of self-esteem, strength, normalcy, inspiration, pride, hope, joy, sense of well-being, & sense of self as a whole woman.

3. Children were important sources of physical, practical, emotional, and social support, and unconditional love to their mothers, buffering the negative effects of HIV.

5. Mothers reported strong physical and psychological attachments to their children, and intensification of the maternal role.

8. Mothers worried about the negative impact of maternal HIV (the illness itself and/or its stigma) on their children, including their negative reactions to it and others' negative reactions to their children.

9. The combination of motherhood and HIV was physically demanding.

10. Maternity/life was often the context for HIV diagnosis/death in women.

14. Mothers struggled with whether to disclose their HIV to their children, worried about the effects of disclosure on child and maternal welfare and the maternal-child relationship, and engaged in strategies to disclose or to delay or avoid disclosing their HIV status to their children.

24. Mothers had special concerns about, hopes for, and were consumed with the health, illness care, future, and placement of HIV+ children.

25. Mothers reported instances, or worried about the negative effects, of HIV– child role reversal, or had adult expectations of their assuming a mother or caretaking role.

(continued)

TABLE 6.4 Four Studies With Largest Intensity Effect Sizes of Findings Pertaining to Motherhood (*Continued*)

Author	Findings	Effect sizes
	27. Sick mothers caring for sick children, the care HIV+ mothers of HIV+ children give them, detracted from their own health and the care of HIV– children.	
	28. Maternal attention and attachment, mother-child relations, and maternal will to live were intensified with an HIV+ child.	
	33. Women had varying knowledge, concerns, and interpretations of, and used various strategies to address, the risk of HIV transmission to fetuses and children.	
	37. Mothers identified self-care as important to being able to live as long as possible to take care of their children, but child care took precedence over maternal self-care.	
	43. Mothers had concerns over child care and/or placement, especially as maternal disease worsened and/or after maternal death.	
	52. Both HIV-related and unrelated factors were involved in women's decisions to conceive, continue, or terminate pregnancies, with the same or different moralities, desires, risk assessments, or circumstances leading to the same or different decisions.	
	53. Women were hurt or angered by providers who offered misinformation, conveyed that they ought not to reproduce, conveyed advice in a hurtful way, or who tried to coerce them concerning reproduction.	

TABLE 6.5 Statements of Findings Contributing to Grounded Theory
of Defensive Motherhood

Ingram, 1996; Ingram et al., 1999a, 2000	HIV+ women face a double bind, by which women are supposed to want motherhood and become mothers, but not if they are HIV+.
	Women struggled with the social ambivalence directed at them as mothers.
	HIV made it hard for women to fulfill the social expectations of mothering.
	Stigma set the stage for defensive mothering.
	Mothers engaged in defensive mothering, which involved strategies to prevent the spread of HIV and stigma, prepare children for a motherless future, and maintain a positive attitude.
	Mothers assumed a defensive posture as they worked to prevent the spread of HIV and its concomitant stigma.
	Preventing the spread of HIV and stigma involved hypervigilant monitoring and the safety work of teaching.
	Mothers taught children about avoiding blood and body fluids and using gloves.
	Mothers taught their children about transmission of HIV through unprotected sexual contact.
	Mothers feared a courtesy stigma directed at their children.
	Mothers monitored the threat posed by the stigma of HIV.
	In spite of advances in the treatment of AIDS, mothers viewed HIV as a death sentence.
	At the heart of the mothers' defensive posture were their defenseless children who faced a motherless future.
	Mothers shared their values with their children.
	Mothers emphasized the importance of loving relationships.
	Mothers taught children about practical topics.
	Mothers felt the temporal urgency of their situation.
	Mothers wrote letters with information for younger children.
	Mothers found it difficult to make custody arrangements for children, especially HIV+ child.
	In spite of widespread anxiety around custody, none of the mothers had legal documentation about their wishes concerning custody of their minor children in the event of their deaths.

(continued)

TABLE 6.5 Statements of Findings Contributing to Grounded Theory of Defensive Motherhood *(Continued)*

Ingram, 1996; Ingram et al., 1999a, 2000 *(cont'd)*	Fear of stigma and its repercussions inhibited mothers from building supportive relationships for their children after their death.
	Although all mothers sought out resources to assist them with legal arrangements for their deaths, none had legal documentation because it was a symbol for giving up and accepting death.
	Mothers sought to leave a positive legacy to their children.
	Most mothers worked to leave special memories about the mother-child relationship in shared experiences, photo albums, video recordings, or written cards and letters.
	The ravages of HIV weakened the mothers' ability to mother physically and emotionally.
	Mothers lived in fear of being discredited as mothers by themselves and others because they were HIV+.
	Mothers worked to strengthen and maintain their mental well-being for their children.
	Children were a reason to live and a focus for life.
	Mothers engaged in strategies to maintain a positive attitude and avoid negativity, including support groups.
	Most mothers spoke of their hopes for a cure, especially mothers of HIV+ children.

TABLE 6.6 Statements of Findings Contributing to Interpretive Explanation of Contribution of Symbolic Capital to HIV-Related Stigma

Grove, Kelly, & Liu, 1997	Women consistently reported that physicians overlooked gynecological manifestations of HIV infection.
	Both physicians and the women themselves suffered from the perceptual block interfering with the diagnostic process embodied in the use of risk group markers. Risk group identification is a common way of (mis)understanding HIV, resulting in delays in diagnosis in individuals who do not fit the risk profile.
	Common themes in women's tales included a past hetero-sexual relationship, an unexplained illness or death, a search for likely causes of symptoms, a final diagnosis after everything else had been ruled out.
	To these mostly heterosexual, White, middle-class women and their physicians, HIV infection was something that happened to "other people."
	A set of contingencies protects the identity and social fate of HIV-seropositive individuals.
	For the women in our sample, obtaining a diagnosis of HIV/AIDS was the first stage of their moral career.
	The second stage of their moral career involved information control and stigma management, the process by which these women attempted to make their lives as normal as possible.
	The women actively segmented their role sets between acquaintances and confidants.
	Their success in segmenting their role sets was dependent upon the fact that no one saw them as belonging to one of the risk groups.
	The strategy most women in our sample followed was selective disclosure.
	Women assessed the consequences of revealing their HIV status to others, and then acted on that assessment.
	Most chose to reveal their HIV status to family and close friends, and to conceal their status from coworkers, neighbors, and other acquaintances.
	Women were afraid that the moral stigma associated with the disease would result in negative consequences, such as losing their job and/or medical benefits or being shunned by coworkers.
	As their illness progressed and absences from work became more frequent, several women continued to conceal their status by using "medical disclaimers," or different disease labels to account for their symptoms, to preserve their moral status.
	The women were able to more easily cover their discreditable status due to the social attributes associated with the symbolic capital they possessed.

(continued)

TABLE 6.6 Statements of Findings Contributing to Interpretive Explanation of Contribution of Symbolic Capital to HIV-Related Stigma *(Continued)*

Grove, Kelly, & Liu *(cont'd)*	Attempts at covering were routinely successful for the women because of their symbolic capital.
	Ironically, much of the success these women had in covering and elective concealment was dependent upon the fact that no one saw them as belonging to one of the risk groups.
	The second role set the women in our study delineated were confidants: primarily family and friends.
	When women made the decision to reveal their HIV status to confidants, normalizing their condition was crucial.
	Disclosure to confidants was always done on a one-to-one basis and involved conscious attempts to manage the meaning of being HIV-seropositive.
	Women with symbolic capital were able to disclose their condition to "safe others," garner sympathy, and continue to have these people in their lives.
	After disclosure, most women continued to receive support and acceptance from family and friends.
	Women were able to elicit sympathy without being marginalized. Their symbolic capital earned them "sympathy credits." They were seen as individuals who merited genuine concern without being sociallyisolated—the fate of many who are discredited.
	The women were stigmatized, but not morally ostracized.
	All but one woman discussed at some length how they were infected: part of their stigma management work. Their stories reflect the prevailing cultural assumption that only certain groups of people are at risk for infection. Disclosure involved not only telling the "facts" about infection but also emphasizing the many nondeviant aspects of their lives.

REFERENCES

Edwards, A., Elwyn, G., Hood, K., & Rollnick, S. (2000). Judging the "weight of evidence" in systematic reviews: Introducing rigor into the qualitative overview stage by assessing signal and noise. *Journal of Evaluation in Clinical Practice, 6,* 177–184.

Edwards, A. G., Russell, I. T., & Stott, N. C. (1998). Signal versus noise in the evidence base for medicine: An alternative to hierarchies of evidence? *Family Practice, 15,* 319–322.

Grove, K. A., Kelly, D. P., & Liu, J. (1997). "But nice girls don't get it": Women, symbolic capital, and the social construction of AIDS. *Journal of Contemporary Ethnography, 26,* 317–337.

Ingram, D. A. (1996). *HIV-positive women: Double binds and defensive mothering.* Unpublished doctoral dissertation, University of Florida, Gainesville.

Ingram, D., & Hutchinson, S. A. (1999). Defensive mothering in HIV-positive mothers. *Qualitative Health Research, 9,* 243–258.

Ingram, D., & Hutchinson, S. A. (2000). Double binds and the reproductive and mothering experiences of HIV-positive women. *Qualitative Health Research, 10,* 117–132.

Onwuegbuzie, A. J. (2003). Effect sizes in qualitative research: A prolegomenon. *Quality & Quantity, 37,* 393–409.

Onwuegbuzie, A. J., & Teddlie, C. (2003). A framework for analyzing data in mixed methods research. In A. Tashakkori & C. Teddlie (Eds.), *Handbook of mixed methods in social and behavioral research* (pp. 351–383). Thousand Oaks, CA: Sage.

Poirier, S., & Ayres, L. (1997). Endings, secrets, and silences: Overreading in narrative inquiry. *Research in Nursing & Health, 20,* 551–557.

Sandelowski, M. (1994). The use of quotes in qualitative research. *Research in Nursing & Health, 17,* 479–482.

Sandelowski, M. (2001). Real qualitative researchers do not count: The use of numbers in qualitative research. *Research in Nursing & Health, 24,* 230–240.

Thorne, S., Jensen, L., Kearney, M. H., Noblit, G., & Sandelowski, M. (2004). Qualitative metasynthesis: Reflections on methodological orientation and ideological agenda. *Qualitative Health Research, 14,* 1342–1365.

Weitz, R. (1993). Powerlessness, invisibility, and the lives of women with HIV disease. *Advances in Medical Sociology, 3,* 101–121.

CHAPTER SEVEN

Synthesizing Qualitative Research Findings:
Qualitative Metasynthesis

You will recall that *qualitative metasynthesis* is an interpretive integration of qualitative findings in primary research reports that are in the form of interpretive syntheses of data: either conceptual/thematic descriptions or interpretive explanations. You have available to you a range of methodological and technical approaches for producing a qualitative metasynthesis of findings in a target domain of study.

APPROACHES TO QUALITATIVE METASYNTHESIS

The term *qualitative metasynthesis* does not by itself signal any one method or technique, or any one way of executing methods or techniques. The approaches you use will depend on the purpose of your project, the product you want to produce, and what the findings in the reports included in your study allow in the way of interpretive treatment. But the end product of qualitative metasynthesis is always an integration of research findings, as opposed to a comparison or critique of them. Here are several approaches to metasynthesis you might use.

Taxonomic Analysis

Taxonomic analysis is an inductive form of domain analysis useful for theory development (Spradley, 1979). Taxonomic analysis has much in common with the axial and selective coding associated with grounded theory (Strauss & Corbin, 1998). In contrast to effect sizes, which show the quantitative range of findings, taxonomies show the conceptual range of findings and provide a foundation for the development of conceptual descriptions and models, theories, or working hypotheses.

Box 7.1 shows a taxonomy we created from the findings extracted pertaining to motherhood in HIV-positive women. In this taxonomy, findings are categorized in two domains—reproductive decision making and the experience of motherhood—by the properties, dimensions, or variations suggested by the findings. Our purpose was not to determine the prevalence of findings—the goal in calculating effect sizes—but rather to identify the underlying conceptual relations signified, albeit not necessarily explicitly expressed, in the findings. The taxonomy is comprised of items that have different "semantic relations" (Spradley, 1979, pp. 117–118) either within the same or between different categories in each domain. For example, the items in the category *reproductive decisions* in the reproductive decision-making domain show an "X-is-a-type-of-Y" relationship (e.g., types of decisions); the items in the category *reproductive outcomes* in the same domain show an "X-is-the-cause/-consequence-of-Y" relationship (e.g., outcomes of the decision to conceive); and the items in the category *justifications* show an "X-is-a-reason-for-doing-Y" relationship (e.g., reasons for having children). The items in the category *types of mothering work* in the experience of motherhood domain show several semantic relations, including "X-is-a-way-to-do-Y" (*surveillance work*), "X-is-a-reason-for-doing-Y" (*information work*), and "X-is-a-cause/-consequence-of-Y" (*accounting work*). Semantic relations are what you see in the findings; they represent an interpretation on your part of how disparate findings are conceptually related to each other.

The variation in semantic relations shown in Box 7.1 reflects our interpretation of the the contexts in which findings appear in the research reports. For example, the dimension of *focus* seemed to us to be the property underlying, and thus the best way to capture, those findings pertaining to what we called *hope work* and *worry work,* whereas the dimensions of *objectives* and *conditions* seemed to capture best the findings pertaining to what we called *legacy work.*

Taxonomic analysis can show not only the theoretical properties of findings explicitly expressed in reports, but also what is not there that ought logically to be there and thereby allow more penetrating syntheses. We included an item in the taxonomy that was called for theoretically by the findings, but was not empirically present in the findings. In the *justifications* category in the domain of reproductive decision making, all of the items refer to justifications "for having" children, which calls for a list of contrasting justifications "for not having" children. Yet no examples of such justifications appeared in the findings. We placed this item in parentheses. We went on to infer from these "missing" findings that although motherhood is for women typically the fulfillment of a cultural norm requiring no justification, it is a deviant act for HIV-positive women requiring justification. Box 7.2 shows another taxonomic analysis of findings pertaining to the management of potentially stigmatizing HIV-related information.

Constant Targeted Comparison

Another analytic device useful for creating metasyntheses of findings is constant targeted comparison. Such comparisons involve the deliberate search for similarities and differences between a target phenomenon and some other extra-study phenomenon (i.e., not addressed in the reports of studies reviewed) with an apparent resemblance to it. The objective in such comparisons is to clarify the defining and overlapping attributes of the target phenomenon in order to minimize the likelihood of inflating its uniqueness and to help discern the relationships between phenomena. This work is similar to the examination of "related cases" in Wilsonian concept analysis (Avant & Abbott, 2000, p. 69) and is a form of constant comparison analysis (Strauss & Corbin, 1998).

In metasynthesis projects, constant targeted comparison entails taking sets of findings as a whole as the target point of comparison, not selected participants' quotations or segments of findings. These comparisons are thus best conducted after you have reduced the findings in all reports into a set of abstracted statements, or represented them in a taxonomy.

You can experiment with comparisons likely best to showcase and penetrate findings. In the case of motherhood in the context of maternal HIV infection, comparisons can be focused on:

(a) *HIV status* (HIV-positive vs. HIV-negative mothers);
(b) *gender* (HIV-positive women/mothers and mothering vs. HIV-positive men/fathers and fathering);
(c) *place of mothering* (at home, homeless shelter, prison);
(d) *procreative status* (HIV-positive childless women vs. HIV-positive mothers);
(e) *type of disease* (mothers with HIV disease vs. mothers with cancer);
(f) *illness characteristics* (maternal HIV infection vs. other maternal chronic, mortal, stigmatizing, and/or transmissible—infectious or genetic—illness);
(g) *race/ethnicity and class* (African American vs. Hispanic vs. Caucasian HIV-positive mothers; middle- vs. working-class HIV-positive mothers); and
(h) *mothers deemed culturally deviant* (mothers in prison or on welfare, adoptive, homeless, lesbian, and teenage mothers).

The use of any one or combinations of these or other objects of comparison has the potential to sharpen and deepen understanding of the common and unique features of motherhood in the context of maternal HIV infection, and of how findings are related to key axes of difference (e.g., gender, race/ethnicity, socioeconomic class, parity, and type of disease). The selection of objects for comparison will depend on your interests and expertise, the nature of the findings themselves, and the state of knowledge about those objects of comparison. Some excellent objects of comparison will not have themselves been the topic of much formal study (e.g., motherhood in the context of chronic illness), and most of these objects will not have been the focus of any integration work because relatively few qualitative research synthesis studies have been conducted.

Constant targeted comparisons will assist you to draw conclusions about the findings in the reports of studies you reviewed and their relationship to other findings. You can show the outcome of this work in narrative form or via visual displays (e.g., a series of Venn diagrams, a conceptual model, a set of working hypotheses).

The following is from Sandelowski & Barroso (2003), and is an example of a narrative presentation of constant targeted comparisons to ascertain the shared and distinctive features of motherhood in the context of maternal HIV infection. The various objects of comparison are italicized.

> Motherhood was central to the identities and lives of HIV-positive women who participated in the studies reviewed, *just as it is to most women who are mothers* (McMahon, 1995). The HIV-positive women studied were *like most women and mothers* in their desire for motherhood, in the opportunities and constraints they perceived as integral to motherhood, and in the work they performed as mothers. HIV infection posed a unique mortal and social threat to these mothers, but their experiences of motherhood clarified and even dramatized *what motherhood typically means and entails for any woman.*
>
> *Like middle- and working-class mothers,* the HIV-positive mothers studied loved their children, worked to protect their lives and to preserve their own capacities and identities as mothers, and found in motherhood an opportunity for self-transformation (i.e., to be better mothers and persons; McMahon, 1995). *Like motherhood for women who have been battered or are addicted to drugs,* motherhood for the HIV-positive women was a source of strength and esteem, an anchor in a turbulent life, and a refuge from and buffer against physical and social adversity (Hardesty & Black, 1999; Irwin, Thorne, & Varcoe, 2002). *Like motherhood for battered women and women with other chronic illnesses and physical disabilities,* though, motherhood for HIV-positive women entailed some impairment of their abilities to perform the physical acts of motherhood and reliance on their children for

instrumental and emotional support (Grue & Laerum, 2002; Thorne, 1990).

Yet unlike other chronic illnesses mothers may have, including potentially mortal and genetically transmissible ones, HIV infection often garners more condemnation than sympathy. Although HIV-positive women share with HIV-positive men the effects of having a stigmatizing illness (Barroso & Powell-Cope, 2000), these effects in women appear paradoxically both intensified and diminished by motherhood. Unlike the primarily gay white men in the Barroso and Powell-Cope study, who found the meaning of their illness in and by themselves, the primarily heterosexual minority women participating in the studies reviewed here found it in motherhood and the care of their children.

But motherhood itself positioned these women precariously between life as a normal woman and life as a deviant one. Motherhood in the context of maternal HIV infection exemplifies the cultural contradictions inherent in Western motherhood, whereby motherhood is both redeeming and damning (Hays, 1996; McMahon, 1995; Thurer, 1994; Weingarten, Surrey, Coll, & Watkins, 1998). Like other marginalized mothers—e.g., in prison, on welfare, and homeless—these HIV-positive women mothered against the odds and could not escape the prevalent idea that they were bad mothers and bad women for even desiring motherhood (Coll, Surrey, & Weingarten, 1998).

Like the mothers on crack cocaine Kearney, Murphy, and Rosenbaum (1994) portrayed, and the addicted mothers Hardesty and Black (1999) described, the HIV-positive mothers in the studies reviewed here sought to maintain their standards for mothering and to avoid becoming or being viewed as bad mothers. The Kearney et al. (1994) explanation of "defensive compensation" (p. 355) as the central process involved in "mothering on crack" shares with virtual motherhood women's desire not only to mother their children well, but to redefine mothering in ways that preserve their identities as good mothers. For the mothers on crack cocaine, the relinquishment of children was considered a form of good mothering. For the HIV-positive mothers, good mothering was also not dependent on being in close physical proximity to children or providing them direct care. For the addicted mothers in the Hardesty and Black study and the HIV-positive mothers in the studies reviewed, just thinking about their children and striving to become good mothers could be construed as good mothering. Although these mothers had sometimes relinquished the care of their children to others, they had not relinquished their claim to motherhood.

Like the physically disabled mothers in the Grue and Laerum (2002) study, the HIV-positive mothers studied found that the discourse of motherhood and of HIV infection were incompatible, the former a discourse of social approbation and inclusion and the latter a discourse of social condemnation and exclusion. Both physically disabled and HIV-positive mothers were not necessarily viewed or treated as mothers, but rather as disabled or infected women. Yet both of these groups of mothers used the discourse of motherhood to negotiate their identities: to draw attention away from their deviant conditions and toward themselves as mothers. *Both of these groups of mothers* worked hard to "pass" as mothers (Grue & Laerum, 2002, p. 678).

Imported Concepts

The depiction of the various activities HIV-positive mothers reportedly performed as *mothering work* is an example of the use of imported concepts to integrate findings. An *imported concept* is one that reviewers borrow from theoretical and empirical literature outside the reports in their projects to integrate—not simply organize—findings. Imported concepts are different from in vivo concepts, or concepts researchers themselves invent from their data to integrate them. We used the sociological concepts of "work" advanced by Strauss and his colleagues (e.g., Corbin & Strauss, 1988; Strauss, Fagerhaugh, Suczek, & Wiener, 1982, 1985; see also, Star, 1995) and of "work object" advanced by Casper (1998). Your selection will depend on your prior knowledge of and sensitization to relevant concepts and theories.

You may also wish to use concepts that researchers themselves imported into their studies to integrate their data. For example, we found that Ingram's (1996) use of the imported psychiatric concept of the "double bind" to interpret the conditions leading to defensive motherhood encompassed well the contradictions of motherhood in the context of maternal HIV infection evident, but not necessarily explicitly expressed in, the findings across reports. The taxonomy in Box 7.1 shows the use of the imported concepts *work* and *work object*. The taxonomy shown in Box 7.2 shows the use of concepts imported from Goffman's classic text on stigma (1993), which also appear in several of the reports reviewed.

Reciprocal Translation and Synthesis of In Vivo and Imported Concepts

Another analytic device useful for creating qualitative metasyntheses of findings is the reciprocal translation and synthesis of in vivo concepts alone or in combination with concepts you import. In contrast to constant targeted comparisons between an in-study phenomenon (i.e., motherhood in the context of maternal HIV infection) and other extra-study phenomena (i.e., motherhood in other contexts), reciprocal translation entails constant comparisons of intra-study conceptual syntheses alone or in combination with concepts you as a reviewer import to integrate findings. The use of reciprocal translation to integrate findings interpretively, as opposed to comparing them interpretively, is an adaptation of meta-ethnography (Noblit & Hare, 1988).

Virtual motherhood is the result of the reciprocal translation and synthesis of one imported concept—Goffman's (1963, p. 19) "virtual identity"—and the five in vivo concepts of "eternal motherhood" (Barnes, Taylor-Brown, & Wiener, 1997), "defensive motherhood" (Ingram, 1996; Ingram & Hutchinson, 1999, 2000), "la protectora," or protective motherhood (Valdez, 1999, 2001), "redefined motherhood" (Van Loon, 2000), and "redefining treatment" (Santacroce, Deatrick, & Ledlie, 2002). Because they represent researchers' interpretive syntheses of data, these concepts lend themselves to metasynthesis by reciprocal translation, whereby reviewers focus on the in vivo concepts, metaphors, or other such interpretive devices researchers used to synthesize their data to determine whether and how they can be translated and integrated into each other. The statements of findings contributing to each of the intra-report syntheses of data are shown in Table 7.1.

The following example from Sandelowski & Barroso (2003) illustrates the reciprocal translation and synthesis process. The key concepts are italicized.

Eternal and redefined motherhood share HIV-positive women's efforts to fulfill what they perceived to be the norms of good mothering even when they were physically unable to fulfill them. *Eternal motherhood* signifies mothering after maternal death. Via the videotapes they created for their children, the HIV-positive mothers in the Barnes et al. study (1997) hoped to create a lasting mothering presence. If not present in the flesh, they were eternally present on videotape. Van Loon's (2000) *redefined motherhood* captures a similar effort by HIV-positive women to bypass the physical requirements of motherhood. In her study, HIV-positive mothers were physically unable to care for their children because the severity of their disease or substance abuse had forced them to relinquish the care or custody of their children to others. Like mothers who have died, mothers separated from their children are also not in physical proximity to them and therefore cannot directly care for their children. In the Santacroce et al. (2002) study, the desire to compensate for transmitting HIV to their children and societal views of motherhood and HIV led mothers to protect their HIV-positive children by continually *redefining the nature and boundaries of treatment* of the child.

The Ingram (1996) and Ingram and Hutchinson (1999, 2000) concept of *defensive motherhood* and Valdez' (1999) "la protectora" (a depiction of HIV-positive Hispanic women as protective mothers) encompass HIV-positive women's efforts to protect their children from contracting HIV and from suffering the effects of the stigma associated with HIV, and to prolong the lives and maximize the quality of lives of their HIV-positive children. Like Ingram's (1996) *defensive mother*, Valdez' (1999) *protective mother* is defending her children against the mortal and social consequences of HIV infection.

A reciprocal translation that embraces the in vivo concepts of eternal, redefined, defensive, and protective motherhood is virtual motherhood. Virtual motherhood conceptually brings together all of the circumstances in which the HIV-positive mothers who participated in the studies reviewed were physically separated from their children (by death, imprisonment, and care or custody arrangements), or otherwise unable to perform as good mothers. The deficits they perceived in their maternal performance generated diverse activities (e.g., creating material mementos for their children, seeking reconciliation with children poorly mothered in the past) to remain mothers to their children and to preserve their own as well as their children's image of themselves as good mothers. Virtual motherhood is the kind of motherhood that can transcend the mortal body and any presumed sins of the flesh.

Virtual motherhood also encompasses Goffman's notion of "*virtual identity*" (1963, p. 19). Goffman referred to the discrepancy that exists between stigmatized persons' actual identity—the one they possess by virtue of some culturally deviant condition—and virtual identity, or the normal or culturally prescribed identity they would ordinarily have and to which they aspire. HIV-positive mothers' efforts to preserve their identities as good mothers are a response to what Ingram (1996) and Ingram and Hutchinson (2000) referred to as the "double bind" of motherhood in the context of maternal HIV infection, whereby HIV-positive women fulfill the cultural mandate for all women to become mothers, but find that the very act of fulfilling it leads to further stigmatization. Having actual identities as "bad" and "guilty" women in large part because they chose to become mothers (and thereby to risk transmitting infection to their "good" and "innocent" children), they struggled to achieve or preserve virtual identities as good mothers.

Virtual motherhood encompasses both embodied and transcendent maternal practices focused on self-care and child care. Motherhood was a highly embodied practice when these mothers worked to stay alive and well for their children, and to protect their children against the mortal and social threat HIV infection posed. Yet the inability to meet the physical requirements of motherhood (in large part because of the physical demands of the infection itself) caused HIV-positive mothers to conceive of motherhood as a disembodied and transcendent practice. Virtual motherhood was a discursive response to all of the circumstances in which the HIV-positive mothers studied were, or anticipated being, physically incapacitated or separated from their children by illness, care and custody arrangements, imprisonment, or death. In order to bypass the physical requirements of motherhood, the HIV-positive mothers recast it as not necessarily demanding direct physical contact with, but rather oversight of, children. Motherhood was defined not only as watching children (a direct embodied encounter), but also, in a more disembodied vein, as watching out for them.

In the physical absence of the mother, motherhood can only be accomplished in the virtual sense: by proxy, remotely, or at a distance. In the social presence of stigma, HIV-positive mothers' identities as mothers remain virtual as long as they are primarily viewed as diseased women. Accordingly, women sought to create mementos and memories to ensure that their children would forever remember them as present, healthy, and good. Even if not present in the flesh, they could always be present in the minds and hearts of their children. Virtual motherhood signifies visions of life and afterlife able to transcend the mortal body and any presumed sins of the flesh, in which children are never motherless, mothers are never childless, and mothers are always good. In virtual motherhood, HIV-positive women found both a reason to live and a way to live forever.

Event Timeline

Another device you may find useful in synthesizing qualitative research findings is the event timeline. Event timelines draw from event analysis and other ethnographic and narrative techniques directed toward delineating and temporally linking selected events (Happ, Swigart, Tate, & Crighton, 2004; Sandelowski, 1999). By placing events of interest to you in temporal relation to each other, you may be able better to see the discrete events constituting the target event or to discern the varied roles events can play—within one report and across reports—as independent, dependent, moderating, and mediating variables. To create event timelines, you will have to track every relation depicted between two or more target events regardless of the number of reports in which it appears or the number of research participants showing this relation. Only after all temporal linkages have been accounted for will you be in a position to ascertain the relative strength of the linkages depicted.

For example, we became interested in ascertaining the relationship between substance abuse and HIV infection after we noted how often substance abuse appeared in the findings of reports of studies conducted with HIV-positive women (for the full report of this analysis, see Barroso & Sandelowski, 2004). In 74 of the 114 reports of studies with HIV-positive women we reviewed, HIV infection and substance abuse recurrently appeared as intersecting events (Ciambrone, 2001), even though substance abuse was the explicit research focus in only two of these reports. (This illustrates another reason the search strategy in qualitative research synthesis studies must initially be inclusive and broad. Findings concerning target events will often be contained in reports of studies that did not have those events as their foci. See chapter 3.) We subsequently searched each of these reports for findings pertaining to substance abuse with a view toward ascertaining how it intersected with HIV infection in the women studied.

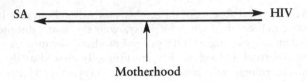

FIGURE 7.1 Illustration of temporal relation of events.

We found that substance abuse (SA) appeared as both a contributor to HIV infection (HIV) and as an outcome of it. SA led to HIV by way of contaminated needles in cases of injection drug use, and by way of sexual relations with an infected partner (either paid relations to support a drug habit or relations under the influence of drugs that contributed to women's reduced capacity to refuse sexual relations or to negotiate the use of condoms). HIV, in turn, appeared as both a contributor to and an outcome of SA. HIV led to the continuation or intensification of prior SA or the initiation of SA (to dull the fear of the diagnosis), and HIV was the result of SA by virtue of the exposure mechanisms described previously. Moreover, the influence of HIV on SA appeared to be mediated by motherhood. Especially in substance-abusing mothers, the diagnosis of HIV infection was the trigger event leading to serious efforts to stop using drugs. These relations can be summarized in Figure 7.1.

Conclusion

The techniques you use interpretively to integrate the findings of qualitative research are as varied as qualitative research itself. Qualitative metasynthesis entails leaps of imagination that you try to communicate as best you can.

BOX 7.1 Taxonomy of Findings Pertaining to Motherhood

I. Reproductive Decision Making

A. Reproductive decisions
  1. Whether to conceive
  2. Whether to continue pregnancy
  3. Whether to terminate pregnancy
B. Reproductive outcomes of reproductive decision making
  1. Decision to conceive
    a. Pregnancy achieved via deliberate efforts
    b. Pregnancy achieved by accident
    c. No pregnancy achieved
  2. Decision not to conceive
    a. Pregnancy avoided or prevented by deliberate efforts
    b. Pregnancy avoided by accident
    c. Accidental pregnancy
  3. Continuation of pregnancy
    a. Live birth
    b. Spontaneous loss
  4. Termination of pregnancy
C. Factors influencing reproductive decision making
  1. HIV-related
    a. Concern over transmission of infection
      a1. Beliefs concerning safety and effectiveness of AZT
        a1a. Positive beliefs
        a1b. Negative beliefs
    b. Health of mother
    c. Concern for child after maternal death
    d. Previous experience with HIV+ child
    e. Health care providers' counsel
  2. Not HIV-related
    a. Importance of motherhood to fulfillment as woman
    b. Completeness of family
    c. Attitude toward and/or availability of abortion
      c1. Stage of pregnancy
    d. Family and/or other women's counsel
    e. Faith and religion
    f. Previous experience with sick child, or child who died
D. Justifications
  1. For having children
    a. Reference to other
      a1. Other HIV+ women have healthy or seroconverted babies
      a2. Drug therapy reduces risk of having HIV+ baby
      a3. God will protect child from harm
      a4. God allowing pregnancy means that having a baby is right
    b. Reference to self
      b1. Already have one healthy baby
      b2. Still young and healthy
      b3. Better able to care for child now than before
  2. For not having children

E. Framework for reproductive decision making
  1. Time
    a. Present-oriented
    b. Future-oriented
  2. Focus
    a. Child-centered
    b. Woman-centered
  3. Nature of moral reasoning
    a. Contextual (ethic of care)
    b. Absolute (ethic of justice)
  4. Agent
    a. God
    b. Self
      b1. By choice
      b2. By default
      b3. By right

II. Experience of Motherhood

A. Impact of motherhood on HIV
  1. Positive impact
    a. Impetus to live
    b. Impetus to self-care
    c. Symptoms improved
    d. Coping improved
    e. Diagnosis of HIV infection
    f. Diminution of stigmatizing and/or mortal effects of HIV
      f1. Children are main or only sources of social support
      f2. Children are legacies, final acts of creation
      f3. Children are sources of self-esteem, pride, power, joy, hope
  2. Negative impact
    a. Intensification of physical burdens of HIV
    b. Aggravation of symptoms
    c. Impaired coping
    d. Exposure of HIV status
      d1. Via inability of children to keep secrets
      d2. Via presence of HIV+ child
    e. Intensification of stigmatizing effects of HIV
      e1. Third arm of "triple stigma"
B. Impact of HIV on motherhood
  1. Positive impact
    a. Impetus to be a better mother
      a1. To enhance already good mother-child relations
      a2. To repair damaged mother-child relations
    b. Impetus to seek medical/prenatal/drug rehabilitation care
  2. Negative impact
    a. Shorter time to mother with "death sentence" of HIV
    b. Imposition of deviant status on motherhood
    c. Impaired maternal/child relations
      c1. Overly intense or enmeshed relations
      c2. Conflicted or estranged relations

         c3. Maternal role confusion
         c4. Child role reversal
     d. Feelings of remorse and/or inadequacy as a mother
     e. Barrier to self-care
     f. Barrier to seeking medical/prenatal care
     g. Impediment to child care
     h. Intensification of physical burdens of motherhood
     i. Offsets joy and life-affirmation of pregnancy and children

C. Mothering work
  1. Conditions for mothering work
     a. Age of child
          a1. Too young for . . .
          a2. Old enough for . . .
     b. HIV status of child
          b1. HIV+ child
          b2. HIV– child
     c. Maternal health status
          c1. Healthy, asymptomatic, not visibly ill
          c2. Sick, symptomatic, visibly ill
     d. Temporal orientation
          d1. Present
          d2. Future
     e. Socioeconomic position of mother
          e1. Advantaged
          e2. Disadvantaged
     f. Ethnic/racial position of mother
          f1. Majority
          f2. Minority
     g. Relations with health care and social service providers
          g1. Positive relations
              g1a. Facilitate utilization of health and social services
              g1b. Facilitate use of AZT
              g1c. Facilitate positive attitude toward self as mother
          g2. Negative relations
              g2a. Impede utilization of health care and social services
              g2b. Impede use of AZT
              g2c. Impede positive attitude toward self as mother
     h. Access to and utilization of health care and social services
          h1. Sufficient
          h2. Insufficient
  2. Objects of mothering work
     a. The medical body (Medical/physical aspects of HIV)
     b. The social body (Stigmatizing effects of HIV)
     c. HIV– child
     d. HIV+ child
     e. Self as mother
  3. Objectives of mothering work
     a. Protection of children
     b. Preservation of identity as good mother
  4. Types of mothering work

a. Surveillance work
  a1. Monitoring spread of HIV to children
  a2. Monitoring spread of HIV-related stigma to children
b. Safety work
  b1. Preventing spread of HIV to children
  b2. Preventing spread of HIV-related stigma to children
c. Information work
  c1. Obtaining information
    c1a. To make mothering decisions
    c1b. To manage HIV+ child's illness
    c1c. For comfort
  c2. Managing information
    c2a. Concerning maternal HIV status
    c2b. Concerning child HIV status
d. Accounting work
  d1. Calculating the risks/benefits of disclosure of maternal or child HIV status
    d1a. Risks/benefits of disclosing maternal HIV to children
      d1a1. To well-being of children
      d1a2. To self as mother
      d1a3. To maternal-child relations
    d1b. Risks/benefits of disclosing maternal HIV to others
      d1b1. To self as mother
      d1b2. To well-being of children
    d1c. Risks/benefits of disclosing child HIV to others
      d1c1. To self as mother
      d1c2. To well-being of HIV+ child
      d1c3. To well-being of HIV– child
    d1d. Risks/benefits of disclosing child HIV to HIV– siblings & other family
      d1d1. To well-being of HIV+ child
      d1d2. To well-being of HIV– child
      d1d3. To sibling & family relations
      d1d4. To self as mother
    d1e. Risks of disclosure in the maternal-child context
      d1e1. Diminished support for child care
      d1e2. Discrimination
      d1e3. Declining maternal and child health
      d1e4. Impaired maternal-child relations
      d1e5. Impaired sibling & family relations
    d1f. Benefits of disclosure in maternal-child context
      d1f1. Support for child care
      d1f2. Special services
      d1f3. Improved maternal and child health
      d1f4. Improved maternal-child relations
      d1e5. Improved sibling & family relations
  d2. Calculating the risks & benefits of taking ARV/AZT in pregnancy, or giving AZT to child
    d2a. Risks of taking or giving ARV/AZT
      d2a1. To self

    d2a1a. Impaired maternal health
    d2a1b. Self-image as "bad" mother
   d2a2. To fetus/infant
    d2a2a. Declining health, death
  d2b. Benefits of taking or giving ARV/AZT
   d2b1. To self
    d2b1a. Preservation of self-/other-identity as
     "good" mother
   d2b2. To fetus/infant
    d2b2a. Improved health
  d2c. Risks of not taking or giving ARV/AZT
   d2c1. To self
    d2c1a. Difficulty obtaining other health services
    d2c1b. Loss of self-/other-identity as "good"
     mother
   d2c2. To fetus/infant
    d2c2a. Difficulty obtaining other health services
    d2c2b. Declining health, death
  d2d. Benefits of not taking or giving ARV/AZT
   d2d1. To self
    d2d1a. Preservation of self-image as "good"
     mother
   d2d2. To fetus/infant
    d2d2a. Maintenance of current health status
 d3. Calculating the risks/benefits of maternal-child health care
  d3a. Risks of seeking or obtaining care
   d3a1. Exposure of HIV
   d3a2. Exposure to persons with advanced disease
   d3a3. Poor treatment by providers
  d3b. Benefits of seeking or obtaining care
   d3b1. Improved maternal & child health
   d3b2. Social support
  d3c. Risks of not seeking or obtaining care
   d3c1. HIV not diagnosed
   d3c2. Declining maternal & child health
  d3d. Benefits of not seeking or obtaining care
   d3d1. HIV not exposed
e. Hope work
 e1. Focus
  e1a. That susceptible child will be seronegative
  e1b. That children will have a good life
  e1c. That there will be a cure for AIDS
  e1d. That they will accomplish mothering goals
f. Worry work
 f1. Focus
  f1a. About the impact of maternal HIV on children
  f1b. About the care of children after maternal death
  f1c. About infecting children
  f1d. About quality of life for children
g. Reconciliation work

      g1. Focus

         g1a. With children not in mother's own care or custody

         g1b. With children poorly mothered in the past

h. Legacy work

    h1. Objectives

       h1a. Preparing children for motherless future

          h1a1. Creation of tangible mementos for child

          h1a2. Providing advice for living and avoiding HIV
               infection

          h1a3. Securing care for child after maternal death

       h1b. Preserving maternal identity while sick and after death

          h1b1. Securing child's image of mother as well and good

          h1b2. Securing self-image as a good mother

    h2. Conditions

       h2a. Time since diagnosis

       h2b. Severity of symptoms

       h2c. Maternal readiness

i. Redefinition work

    i1. Focus

       i1a. Mothering

          i1a1. To include mothering that fails to conform to cul-
               tural norms

          i1a2. To include mothering of child not in maternal care
               or custody

          i1a3. To include mothering after maternal death

       i1b. Illness situation

          i1b1. Maintaining a positive attitude for children

          i1b2. Viewing HIV infection as an opportunity

j. Body work

    j1. Focus

       j1a. Physical aspects of maternal HIV

       j1b. Physical aspects of child's HIV

       j1c. Physical aspects of everyday child care

k. Grief work

    k1. Focus

       k1a. Loss of child

BOX 7.2 Taxonomy of Findings Pertaining to HIV-Related Information Management

A. Framework for information management
   a. Who will tell
   b. Whom to tell
   c. When to tell (time)
      i.   Immediately after diagnosis
      ii. Delayed until adjust to diagnosis
      iii. Before imminent disclosure by others
      iv. Any opportune moment
   d. When to tell (necessary circumstance)
      i.   A need to know exists
      ii.   A right to know exists
      iii. A physical & emotional capacity or readiness to tell exists (in the HIV+ woman)
      iv.   A physical & emotional capacity or readiness to know exists (in the target of disclosure)
      v.   Transmission of HIV infection is likely
      vi.   Target of disclosure is trustworthy
      vii. Target of disclosure can keep a secret
      viii. Risk of rejection or harm to self is low
      ix.   Risk of harm to, or burden of knowing for, beloved others is low (courtesy stigma)
   e. What to tell
      i.   Everything
      ii. Something
      iii. Nothing
   f. Why to tell
      i.   To obtain health and social services
      ii. To secure social support
      iii. To prevent transmission of infection
      iv. To prevent mismanaged disclosure
      v.   To maintain certain identities
      vi. To disavow certain identities
   g. Why not to tell
      i.   To obtain health and social services
      ii. To preserve social support
      iii. To prevent discrimination
      iv. To prevent suffering and burden of loved ones (courtesy stigma)
      v.   To fulfill wishes of family members to maintain secrecy
      vi. To maintain certain identities & in-group alignments
      vii. To disavow certain identities & out-group alignments
B. Managed disclosure & concealment
   a. Full disclosure
   b. Partial or selective disclosure or concealment
      i. Covering
   c. Full concealment
      i. Passing
      ii. Lying

      iii.   Keeping silent
      iv.   Circumventing need to disclose
C. Mismanaged disclosure & concealment
  a. Disclosure by undesignated agent
  b. Discrediting clues & cues
  c. Unwanted serial disclosures

TABLE 7.1 Statements of Findings Contributing to Intra-Report Conceptual Syntheses of Data

Author, Conceptual synthesis	Statements of findings constituting conceptual synthesis
Barnes et al., 1997 *Eternal motherhood*	Videotapes are a means to leave a legacy to children.
	Mothers choose how they will present themselves.
	These videotaped legacies are stories in which they give gendered advice, disclose personal secrets, and express guilt.
	The concept contextualizing these stories is "eternal mothering."
	Mothers in this study warn their children about how to avoid mistakes the mothers had made, emphasizing the role gender played in their lives and how it shaped their choices and regrets and therefore warnings.
	Mothers warn their noninfected children about AIDS as a deadly disease.
	The disclosure of HIV/AIDS was not the primary secret shared by the mothers.
	Mothers demonstrated a concern that by disclosing their HIV status they might be transferring the potential stigmatization associated with HIV/AIDS to their children.
	Some women reported that telling their HIV status to their children face to face was one of the most difficult parts of the disease process.
	Universal to mothers is the guilt for not being the ideal mother as defined by themselves, and their perception of cultural expectations.
	Mothers addressed their guilt for their mothering, and the stigma associated with AIDS.
	Mothers attempted to diminish the negative impact of their HIV/AIDS status and life choices and to free their children from feeling shame.
	Most mothers express regrets about aspects of their mothering.
	There is an eternal aspect of their mothering characterized by anticipating future events, giving advice for life, and promising to be eternally available in spirit, even after their physical death.
	Eternal mothering, as embodied in videotapes, means mothering does not end at maternal death.
Synthesized finding	*Eternal motherhood*: Eternal aspects of motherhood were characterized by anticipating future events, giving advice for life, and promising to be eternally available in spirit, even after physical death.

(continued)

TABLE 7.1 Statements of Findings Contributing to Intra-Report Conceptual Syntheses of Data *(Continued)*

Author, Conceptual synthesis	Statements of findings constituting conceptual synthesis
Ingram, 1996; Ingram et al., 1999a, 2000	HIV+ women face a double bind, by which women are supposed to want motherhood and become mothers, but not if they are HIV+.
Defensive motherhood	Women struggled with the social ambivalence directed at them as mothers.
	HIV made it hard for women to fulfill the social expectations of mothering.
	Stigma set the stage for defensive mothering.
	Mothers engaged in defensive mothering, which involved strategies to prevent the spread of HIV and stigma, prepare children for a motherless future, and maintain a positive attitude.
	Mothers assumed a defensive posture as they worked to prevent the spread of HIV and its concomitant stigma.
	Preventing the spread of HIV and stigma involved hypervigilant monitoring and the safety work of teaching.
	Mothers taught children about avoiding blood and body fluids and using gloves.
	Mothers taught their children about transmission of HIV through unprotected sexual contact.
	Mothers feared a courtesy stigma directed at their children.
	Mothers monitored the threat posed by the stigma of HIV.
	In spite of advances in the treatment of AIDS, mothers viewed HIV as a death sentence.
	At the heart of the mothers' defensive posture were their defenseless children who faced a motherless future.
	Mothers shared their values with their children.
	Mothers emphasized the importance of loving relationships.
	Mothers taught children about practical topics.
	Mothers felt the temporal urgency of their situation.
	Mothers wrote letters with information for younger children.
	Mothers found it difficult to make custody arrangements for children, especially an HIV+ child.

TABLE 7.1 *(Continued)*

Author, Conceptual synthesis	Statements of findings constituting conceptual synthesis
	In spite of widespread anxiety around custody, none of the mothers had legal documentation about their wishes concerning custody of their minor children in the event of their deaths.
	Fear of stigma and its repercussions inhibited mothers from building supportive relationships for their children after their death.
	Although all mothers sought out resources to assist them with legal arrangements for their deaths, none had legal documentation because they were a symbol for giving up and accepting death.
	Mothers sought to leave a positive legacy to their children.
	Most mothers worked to leave special memories about the mother-child relationship in shared experiences, photo albums, video recordings, or written cards and letters.
	The ravages of HIV weakened the mothers' ability to mother physically and emotionally.
	Mothers lived in fear of being discredited as mothers by themselves and others because they were HIV+.
	Mothers worked to strengthen and maintain their mental well-being for their children.
	Children were a reason to live and a focus for life.
	Mothers engaged in strategies to maintain a positive attitude and avoid negativity, including support groups.
	Most mothers spoke of their hopes for a cure, especially mothers of HIV+ children.
Synthesized finding	*Defensive motherhood*: Faced with a double bind, by which women are supposed to want motherhood and become mothers, but not if they are HIV+, mothers engaged in defensive mothering, which involved strategies to prevent the spread of HIV and stigma, prepare children for a motherless future, and maintain a positive attitude.
Valdez, 1999 *Protective motherhood*	Pregnancy and children became the impetus that appeared to take the women to "Ofrecer."
	Ofrecer is "an offer to change," and is characterized by a woman's negotiating with God on behalf of her child.
	The Hispanic woman during the Ofrecer stage promises to do good, namely live for her child and reveal her status to benefit others.

(continued)

TABLE 7.1 Statements of Findings Contributing to Intra-Report Conceptual Syntheses of Data *(Continued)*

Author, Conceptual synthesis	Statements of findings constituting conceptual synthesis
	Her exchange is not for herself, or for more time, but for the life of her child.
	Despite lack of disclosure to children, most women had made arrangements for their children after their death.
	Most women left significant family members with detailed instructions on the disposition of the children. Other women wrote lengthy letters to each of their children, to be given to them upon their death.
	Other women hoped that they would live long enough to let their children grow to more of an acceptable age to tolerate the news.
	Some of the women expressed more fear of disclosure for their children and families.
	Day-to-day, women cared for families while struggling with their own physical and emotional well-being.
	Women's strength to live came partly from being mothers.
	Women saw their lives as important because they had to care for their children and their families.
	When faced with death, women chose the path of living for their child rather than accepting to die.
	Their decision to live and emerge as La Protectora was influenced by the birth of their child and the revelation of the child's negative status.
Synthesized finding	*Protective motherhood*: "La Protectora" is an intensification of the mother role following diagnosis of HIV infection, in which women bargain for the life and health of their children.
Van Loon, 2000 *Redefined motherhood*	All but one of the women reported that motherhood was their most important role.
	Mothers recognized difficulties in child-rearing and relationships with children due to HIV.
	Mothers focused greater attention on the benefits of having children and the supportive functions served by the children.
	Despite changes in physical status due to AIDS, most mothers continued acting as caregivers to their children.
	When physical decline hindered their ability to perform certain functions associated with motherhood, or when their children no longer lived with them, women redefined the role of mother.

TABLE 7.1 *(Continued)*

Author, Conceptual synthesis	Statements of findings constituting conceptual synthesis
	By altering the meaning of motherhood, they were able to retain the role and the status and satisfaction it provided.
	The women defined the role of mother broadly to include education, emotional support, discipline, physical care, involvement in the children's activities, and financial responsibility.
	Mothering was affected by both changes in health status and issues unique to AIDS.
	Changing health status made some tasks associated with motherhood more difficult to perform, particularly those involving physical exertion.
	Mothers also had to negotiate special concerns associated with AIDS, such as stigma and isolation, ways their illness might affect their children's well-being, and the impact of widespread loss in the family's social network.
	Mothers tried to protect their children from HIV-related stigma.
	Mothers tried to prevent isolation of their children.
	Mothers knew that living with a sick mother could be emotionally troubling for children.
	The effect of widespread loss due to AIDS was another concern for these mothers.
	Mothers reported frustration and difficulties in dealing with their children.
	But the benefits of motherhood outweighed the burdens.
	Mothers looked to their children for practical help, emotional support, and, most important, motivation.
	Changing health status limited role performance for some mothers and had already resulted in placement of their children with others.
	All mothers were aware that others would need to assume responsibility for their children if they died and had thought about plans for their children's future.
	Most mothers had plans in progress, either making informal arrangements with relatives or working with agencies to formalize future adoptions.
	To retain the maternal role in the face of threats to motherhood, mothers redefined motherhood, emphasizing tasks that could be maintained despite changing health status and, when those tasks could no longer be performed, reframing the role of mother as one of oversight of children's well-being.

(continued)

TABLE 7.1 Statements of Findings Contributing to Intra-Report Conceptual Syntheses of Data *(Continued)*

Author, Conceptual synthesis	Statements of findings constituting conceptual synthesis
	Drug-abusing women struggled to define relationships with children who had been placed out of the home.
	Mothers reported troubled relationships with adult children.
	Troubled relations with adult children appeared in women with drug-use histories whose children had been neglected earlier in their lives, and in women who were emotionally closer to younger children because of the constraints of their illness.
Synthesized finding	*Redefined motherhood:* To retain the maternal role in the face of threats to motherhood, mothers redefined motherhood, emphasizing tasks that could be maintained despite changing health status and, when those tasks could no longer be performed, reframing the role of mother as one of oversight of children's well-being.
Santacroce et al., 2002 *Redefining treatment*	The women knew the harm associated with HIV and, as mothers, wanted to protect their children from being similarly harmed.
	Mothers' behaviors were motivated by desires to compensate for causing the disease and transmitting HIV to their children.
	Women believed that a way to protect their children with HIV from additional hurt was to protect their children's emotions.
	Women protected emotions by highlighting their maternal virtues and concern for their children rather than emphasizing their histories of engagement in risk behaviors that placed them and their children in the path of HIV.
	Mothers' beliefs about protective mothering seemed to originate from the importance they placed on the maternal role, as well as society's views about mothers, injection drug use, and persons with HIV.
	The women seemed acutely aware of society's views regarding persons with HIV; they once held those views themselves.
	The basic psychosocial problem that HIV presented to mothers was protecting their children from the harm the mothers associated with the condition.
	The central process that explained how mothers protected their children was conceptualized as redefining treatment, referring to the cognitive and

TABLE 7.1 *(Continued)*

Author, Conceptual synthesis	Statements of findings constituting conceptual synthesis
	behavioral changes that occurred in mothers from the time their children's diagnosis was declared until an unknown period in the course of HIV.
	At first, mothers believed they could prevent or indefinitely delay HIV-related harm to their children.
	Over time, as mothers experienced changes in their children's condition and other concerns or supports, mothers' definitions of harm and treatments changed.
	Mothers' initial hopes evolved, and their ideas about treatment were reformulated in terms of goals and strategies to fit the reality of a progressive and inevitably fatal illness occurring within a highly developed medical treatment context.
Synthesized finding	*Redefining treatment*: Form of protective motherhood whereby the desire to compensate for transmitting HIV and societal views of motherhood and HIV led women to protect HIV+ children by continually redefining the nature and boundaries of treatment.

REFERENCES

Avant, K. C., & Abbott, C. A. (2000). Wilsonian concept analysis: Applying the technique. In B. L. Rodgers & K. A. Knafl (Eds.), *Concept development in nursing: Foundations, techniques, and applications* (2nd ed., pp. 65–76). Philadelphia: W. B. Saunders.

Barnes, D. B., Taylor-Brown, S., & Wiener, L. (1997). "I didn't leave y'all on purpose": HIV-infected mothers' videotaped legacies for their children. *Qualitative Sociology, 20,* 7–32.

Barroso, J., & Powell-Cope, G. M. (2000). Metasynthesis of qualitative research on living with HIV infection. *Qualitative Health Research, 10,* 340–353.

Barroso, J., & Sandelowski, M. (2004). Substance abuse in HIV-positive women. *Journal of the Association of Nurses in AIDS Care, 15(5),* 48–59.

Casper, M. J. (1998). Negotiations, work objects, and the unborn patient: The interactional scaffolding of fetal surgery. *Symbolic Interaction, 21,* 379–400.

Ciambrone, D. A. (2001). Illness and other assaults on self: The relative impact of HIV/AIDS on women's lives. *Sociology of Health & Illness, 23,* 517–540.

Coll, C. G., Surrey, J. L., & Weingarten, K. (Eds.). (1998). *Mothering against the odds: Diverse voices of contemporary mothers.* New York: Guilford Press.

Corbin, J., & Strauss, A. (1988). *Unending work and care: Managing chronic illness at home.* San Francisco: Jossey-Bass.

Goffman, E. (1963). *Stigma: Notes on the management of spoiled identity.* Englewood Cliffs, NJ: Prentice-Hall.

Grue, L., & Laerum, K. T. (2002). "Doing motherhood": Some experiences of mothers with physical disabilities. *Disability & Society, 17,* 671–683.

Happ, M. B., Swigart, V., Tate, J., & Crighton, M. H. (2004). Event analysis techniques. *Advances in Nursing Science, 27(3),* 239–248.

Hardesty, M., & Black, T. (1999). Mothering through addiction: A survival strategy among Puerto Rican addicts. *Qualitative Health Research, 9,* 602–619.

Hays, S. (1996). *The cultural contradictions of motherhood.* New Haven, CT: Yale University Press.

Ingram, D. A. (1996). *HIV-positive women: Double binds and defensive mothering.* Unpublished doctoral dissertation, University of Florida, Gainesville.

Ingram, D., & Hutchinson, S. A. (1999). Defensive mothering in HIV-positive mothers. *Qualitative Health Research, 9,* 243–258.

Ingram, D., & Hutchinson, S. A. (2000). Double binds and the reproductive and mothering experiences of HIV-positive women. *Qualitative Health Research, 10,* 117–132.

Irwin, L. G., Thorne, S., & Varcoe, C. (2002). Strength in adversity: Motherhood for women who have been battered. *Canadian Journal of Nursing Research, 34(4),* 47–57.

Kearney, M. H., Murphy, S., & Rosenbaum, M. (1994). Mothering on crack cocaine: A grounded theory analysis. *Social Science & Medicine, 38,* 351–361.

McMahon, M. (1995). *Engendering motherhood: Identity and self-transformation in women's lives.* New York: Guilford Press.

Noblit, G. W., & Hare, R. D. (1988). *Meta-ethnography: Synthesizing qualitative studies.* Newbury Park, CA: Sage.

Sandelowski, M. (1999). Time and qualitative research. *Research in Nursing & Health, 22,* 79–87.

Sandelowski, M., & Barroso, J. (2003). Motherhood in the context of maternal HIV infection. *Research in Nursing & Health, 26,* 470–482.

Santacroce, S. J., Deatrick, J. A., & Ledlie, L. S. (2002). Redefining treatment: How biological mothers manage their children's treatment for perinatally acquired HIV. *AIDS Care, 14,* 247–260.

Spradley, J. P. (1979). *The ethnographic interview.* Fort Worth, TX: Harcourt Brace Jovanovich.

Star, S. L. (1995). Epilogue: Work and practice in social studies of science, medicine, and technology. *Science, Technology, & Human Values, 20,* 501–507.

Strauss, A., & Corbin, J. (1998). *Basics of qualitative research: Techniques and procedures for developing grounded theory* (2nd ed.). Thousand Oaks, CA: Sage.

Strauss, A., Fagerhaugh, S., Suczek, B., & Wiener, C. (1982). The work of hospitalized patients. *Social Science & Medicine, 16,* 977–986.

Strauss, A., Fagerhaugh, S., Suczek, B., & Wiener, C. (1985). *Social organization of medical work.* Chicago: University of Chicago Press.

Thorne, S. E. (1990). Mothers with chronic illness: A predicament of social construction. *Health Care for Women International, 11,* 209–221.

Thurer, S. (1994). *The myths of motherhood: How culture reinvents the good mother.* New York: Houghton Mifflin.

Valdez, M. D. (1999). *La Protectora (The Protectress): A metaphor for HIV+ Hispanic women.* Unpublished doctoral dissertation, Texas Woman's University, Denton.

Valdez, M. D. (2001). A metaphor for HIV positive Mexican and Puerto Rican women. *Western Journal of Nursing Research, 23,* 517–535.

Van Loon, R. A. (2000). Redefining motherhood: Adaptation to role change for women with AIDS. *Families in Society: The Journal of Contemporary Human Services, 81,* 152–161.

Weingarten, K., Surrey, J. L., Coll, C. G., & Watkins, M. (1998). Introduction. In C. G. Coll, J. L. Surrey, & K. Weingarten (Eds.), *Mothering against the odds: Diverse voices of contemporary mothers* (pp. 1–14). New York: Guilford Press.

CHAPTER EIGHT

Optimizing the Validity of Qualitative Research Synthesis Studies

From the time you conceive your study and throughout its execution, you must always be thinking of ways to optimize the validity of the research synthesis you produce. Because many orientations to validity in qualitative research exist, you will have to clarify and defend for yourself, and then for the audiences for your study, your particular take on validity.

We assume here a realist stance toward validity, by which we mean to convey our effort to maintain truth as a "regulative ideal" (Murphy & Dingwall, 2001, p. 346). For qualitative research synthesis to mean anything in the practice disciplines, reviewers have to maintain a primary commitment to producing "faithful accounts of a 'real' world": if not to big TRUTH, then to a "small(er)-'t' truth" (Michalowski, 1997, p. 67, n. 1). They have to operate "as if truth holds still" (Thorne, Jensen, Kearney, Noblit, & Sandelowski, 2004, p. 1354), at least for awhile. Reviewers maintain contact with the empirical world as depicted in the research reports in their synthesis study, even as they demonstrate their awareness of the series of interpretive acts and discursive practices entailed in any effort to synthesize research findings, the political-ideological contexts of the body of research that is the focus of their study, and of issues involving authority and representation (Alvesson & Sköldberg, 2000, p. 238). Reviewers accept that truth is inescapably socially constructed, but recognize that although multiple versions of truth can exist, multiple contradictory versions of it cannot. And they recognize that validity is itself "a social construction, . . . rhetorical organization of arguments, . . . (and) feat of persuasion" (Aguinaldo, 2004, p. 128).

The mechanisms we feature here to promote valid study procedures and outcomes are directed toward enhancing the descriptive, interpretive, theoretical, and pragmatic validity of research integrations (Kvale, 1995; Maxwell, 1992; Seale, 1999). These mechanisms include: (a) the maintenance of an audit trail (Rodgers & Cowles, 1993); (b) ongoing negotiation of consensual validity (Belgrave & Smith, 1995; Eisner, 1991); and (c) expert peer review (Sandelowski, 1998).

Descriptive validity refers to the factual accuracy of data. In qualitative research synthesis studies, this means the identification of all relevant research reports and the accurate identification and characterization of information from each report included in the study. *Interpretive validity,* the type of validity referred to in descriptions of member checking or respondent validation (e.g., Bloor, 1983), refers to the full and fair representation of actors' understandings or points of view. You will recall that in qualitative research synthesis studies, the actors are the researchers who conducted and authored the reports of the studies included in your project; they are not the participants who were the subjects of study. *Theoretical validity* refers to the credibility of researchers' interpretations. The primary data in qualitative research synthesis studies consist of the findings in reports of the studies in your project. Accordingly, theoretical validity in these studies refers to the credibility of the (a) methods you—as a reviewer—developed to produce your integrations and to the (b) research integrations themselves, or your interpretation of researchers' findings. *Pragmatic validity* refers to the utility and transferability of knowledge. In qualitative research synthesis studies, pragmatic validity refers to the applicability, timeliness, and translatability for practice of the research integrations, or evidence syntheses, you produce.

The descriptive validity of the search and retrieval procedures you use can be addressed by: (a) employing all the major channels of communication and iterative search strategies to ensure an exhaustive search, as described in chapter 3; (b) consultation with reference librarians; (c) having each search conducted by at least two members of the research team trained to conduct exhaustive searches; (d) holding weekly research team meetings to discuss search and retrieval procedures; and (e) using reference manager software, and decision and other tools, to track search outcomes. Both the descriptive and interpretive validity of the appraisal of study reports can be addressed by: (a) having at least two members of the research team complete individual appraisals of every report; (b) holding weekly research team meetings to discuss both the individual and comparative appraisals of reports; and (c) contacting authors of primary study reports whenever the clarification of information in their reports is deemed essential. For example, in our study, we contacted researchers when we were uncertain about the relationships between sets of findings in two or more reports from apparently the same parent study with over-lapping samples. The theoretical and pragmatic validity of the integrations you produce can be addressed by: (a) holding weekly research team meetings in which interpretive techniques are the focus of discussion; (b) consultation with experts in research methods; and (c) having your integrated findings evaluated by research and clinical experts in the target area of study.

AUDIT TRAIL

A key mechanism for optimizing the validity of study procedures and outcomes is the audit trail (Rodgers & Cowles, 1993). This trail will consist of documents tracking search outcomes and the "reflexive accounting" (Seale, 1999, p. 160)—in material form (e.g., databases, narrative text, memos, tabular and other visual displays)—of the procedural and interpretive moves made during the course of your study. The audit trail should include documentation of the strategies used in each phase of your project, and the rationale behind the selection, use, development, or abandonment of those strategies. This documentation is itself treated as data and serves to enhance the credibility of study outcomes by making transparent the series and sequence of judgments made during the life of your study. All team members should have electronic access to shared files that contain all of the individual and collective work of your study.

NEGOTIATED CONSENSUAL VALIDITY

Integral to efforts to address descriptive, interpretive, theoretical, and pragmatic validity is the idea of "negotiated validity" (Belgrave & Smith, 1995). Negotiated validity refers to a social process and goal, especially relevant to collaborative, methodological, and integration research, whereby research team members articulate, defend, and persuade others of the "cogency" or "incisiveness" of their points of view (Eisner, 1991, pp. 112–113), or show their willingness to abandon views that are no longer tenable. The essence of negotiated validity is consensus. This consensus does not rely on unanimity per se as unanimity is often achieved by forcing conformity and often results in simplifications that compromise validity (Eisner, 1991; Hak & Bernts, 1996). Traditional techniques for establishing and demonstrating inter-rater reliability, for example, offer no assurance of truth, but rather only confirmation of the fact that raters can be made to agree. A correlation coefficient is itself a product of a socially negotiated process, an agent that participates in the reproduction of that process, and a rhetorical device in the literary technology known as the empirical research report (Gephart, 1988; Shapin, 1984). Moreover, the place of inter-rater reliability in assessing validity in qualitative research is highly contested (Armstrong, Gosling, Weinman, & Marteau, 1997; Churchill, Lowery, McNally, & Rao, 1998; Weinberger et al., 1998).

Favoring a negotiated consensus over a measured reliability view of validity in integration studies is the variability in assessments of common study elements in research integration studies and the impact of even apparently minor decisions made in the review process on the conclusions drawn. In our study, even intra-reviewer consistency was sometimes difficult to achieve as reviewers saw a deficiency in one report as acceptable but the same deficiency in another report as unacceptable. Most scholars agree that the most important factor optimizing the validity of research integration studies is not the standardization of judgments, but rather the explication of the many judgments required to conduct these studies and to produce research integrations.

Accordingly, your orientation to validity should reside largely in the consensus achieved by negotiation and founded on the clear explanation of judgments. This orientation does not preclude conventional reliability testing, but rather prevents it from becoming the driving force in your study. To facilitate the process of negotiated validity, you and your team (including your consultants) can use a "think aloud" strategy (Fonteyn, Kuipers, & Grobe, 1993) to articulate your reasoning regarding, for example, characterizing studies, determining whether they meet inclusion criteria, identifying their findings, and fitting certain analytic techniques to certain kinds of findings. Reasons for both agreement and disagreement should be explored and disagreements negotiated until a comfortable resolution is reached. The think aloud process, which should also become part of the written audit trail, allows you and your team to not only better understand your own and other members' points of view, but also enhances the reflexivity of teamwork (Barry, Britten, Barber, Bradley, & Stevenson, 1999) essential to valid outcomes in team qualitative and research integration studies.

EXPERT PEER REVIEW

A key mechanism for maximizing theoretical and pragmatic validity is expert peer review whereby the procedures and outcomes of a study are continually subject to scrutiny and critique by persons with the requisite research and clinical knowledge. For example, you can ask experts in qualitative research to apply the appraisal and integration procedures you used to a purposefully selected sample of reports to evaluate their reliability and validity. You can ask clinical experts to transform the integration you produced into a set of usable guidelines for practice. As "translating is the ultimate act of comprehending" (Manguel, 1996, p. 266), you will have a good test of what expert practitioners saw in your findings and of the "utilization value" of these findings (Smaling, 2003, pp. 20–21).

Table 8.1 summarizes the procedures for optimizing the validity of qualitative research synthesis studies. You may wish to add or revise procedures to fit the unique circumstances of your synthesis project.

TABLE 8.1 Procedures to Optimize Validity in Qualitative Research Synthesis Studies

Type of validity	Descriptive	Interpretive	Theoretical	Pragmatic
Procedure				
Use of all search channels of communication	X			
Contact primary study investigators.	X	X		
Consult with reference librarians.	X			
Consult with experts in research synthesis.			X	
Consult with clinical experts.				X
Independent searching by at least two reviewers	X			
Independent appraisal of each report by at least two reviewers	X	X		
Weekly research team meetings to discuss search outcomes and to formulate and refine search strategies	X			
Weekly research team meetings to discuss appraisal outcomes and to formulate and refine study appraisal strategies	X	X		
Weekly research team meetings to establish areas of consensus and to negotiate consensus in areas and cases of dispute	X	X	X	
Documentation (audit trail) of all procedures, changes in procedure, and results; individual and group think aloud sessions	X	X	X	X

REFERENCES

Aguinaldo, J. P. (2004). Rethinking validity in qualitative research from a social constructionist perspective: From "is this valid research?" to "what is this research valid for?" *The Qualitative Report, 9(1)*, 127–136. Retrieved January 5, 2005, from www.nova.edu/ssss/QR/QR9-1/aguinaldo.pdf

Alvesson, M., & Sköldberg, K. (2000). *Reflexive methodology: New vistas for qualitative research.* London: Sage.

Armstrong, D., Gosling, A., Weinman, J., & Marteau, T. (1997). The place of inter-rater reliability in qualitative research: An empirical study. *Sociology, 31,* 597–606.

Barry, C. A., Britten, N., Barber, N., Bradley. C., & Stevenson, F. (1999). Using reflexivity to optimize teamwork in qualitative research. *Qualitative Health Research, 9,* 26–44.

Belgrave, L. L., & Smith, K. J. (1995). Negotiated validity in collaborative ethnography. *Qualitative Inquiry, 1,* 69–86.

Bloor, M. J. (1983). Notes on member validation. In R. M. Emerson (Ed.), *Contemporary field research: A collection of readings* (pp. 156–172). Boston: Little, Brown.

Churchill, S. D., Lowery, J. E., McNally, O., & Rao, A. (1998). The question of reliability in interpretive psychological research: A comparison of three phenomenologically based protocol analyses. In R. Valle (Ed.), *Phenomenological inquiry in psychology: Existential and transpersonal dimensions* (pp. 63–85). New York: Plenum Press.

Eisner, E. W. (1991). *The enlightened eye: Qualitative inquiry and the enhancement of educational practice.* New York: Macmillan.

Fonteyn, M. E., Kuipers, B., & Grobe, S. J. (1993). A description of think aloud method and protocol analysis. *Qualitative Health Research, 3,* 430–441.

Gephart, R. P. (1988). *Ethnostatistics: Qualitative foundations for quantitative research.* Beverly Hills, CA: Sage.

Hak, T., & Bernts, T. (1996). Coder training: Theoretical training or practical socialization? *Qualitative Sociology, 19,* 235–257.

Kvale, S. (1995). The social construction of validity. *Qualitative Inquiry, 1,* 19–40.

Manguel, A. (1996). *A history of reading.* Toronto: Knopf.

Maxwell, J. A. (1992). Understanding and validity in qualitative research. *Harvard Educational Review, 62,* 279–300.

Michalowski, R. J. (1997). Ethnography and anxiety: Field work and reflexivity in the vortex of U.S.-Cuban relations. In R. Hertz (Ed.), *Reflexivity & voice* (pp. 45–69). Thousand Oaks, CA: Sage.

Murphy, E., & Dingwall, R. (2001). The ethics of ethnography. In P. Atkinson, A. Coffey, S. Delamont, J. Lofland, & L. Lofland (Eds.), *Handbook of ethnography* (pp. 339–351). London: Sage.

Rodgers, B. L., & Cowles, K. V. (1993). The qualitative research audit trail: A complex collection of documentation. *Research in Nursing & Health, 16,* 219–226.

Sandelowski, M. (1998). The call to experts in qualitative research. *Research in Nursing & Health, 21,* 467–471.

Seale, C. (1999). *The quality of qualitative research.* London: Sage.

Shapin, S. (1984). Pump and circumstance: Robert Boyle's literary technology. *Social Studies of Science, 14,* 481–520.

Smaling, A. (2003). Inductive, analogical, and communicative generalization. *International Journal of Qualitative Methods, 2*(1). Article 5. Retrieved September 22, 2003, from http://www.ualberta.ca/~ijqm/backissues/2_1/html/smaling.html

Thorne, S., Jensen, L., Kearney, M. H., Noblit, G., & Sandelowski, M. (2004). Qualitative meta-synthesis: Reflections on methodological orientation and ideological agenda. *Qualitative Health Research, 14,* 1342–1365.

Weinberger, M., Ferguson, J. A., Westmoreland, G., Mamlin, L. A., Segar, D. S., Eckert, G. J., et al. (1998). Can raters consistently evaluate the content of focus groups? *Social Science & Medicine, 46,* 929–933.

CHAPTER NINE

Presenting Syntheses
of Qualitative
Research Findings

As soon as you have an idea of the lines of integration you want to pursue, you are ready to consider the form in which it might be disseminated. Even though we separate them here, content and form—and analysis, interpretation, and representation—are inseparable in qualitative research and, therefore, in qualitative research synthesis. Essential to these processes are putting ideas into material form on paper or on screen. In qualitative research, writing and other forms of embodying ideas—such as tables, graphs, diagrams, drawings, and photos—are modes, not merely end products, of inquiry (Richardson, 2000).

In this chapter, we address issues related to the dissemination of and representation in qualitative research. We offer you ideas for presenting the results of your integration studies in ways that accommodate them to the publication venues to which you are submitting your report but do not compromise your study or qualitative inquiry.

WRITING AND REPRESENTATION

The effort to write up the results of a qualitative research synthesis study will inevitably compel you to address the challenges of representation in qualitative studies. As we first noted in the introduction, such studies always raise issues concerning who and what is being represented in reports of qualitative research synthesis.

In the mid-1980s, ethnographers began to address what has come to be known as the "crisis of representation" (Denzin & Lincoln, 2000,

p. 16; Lincoln & Denzim, 2000, p. 1050) in anthropology, by which they meant the recognition of the ethics, politics, and even hubris involved in anthropologists' efforts to portray the lives of "Others." These and other researchers began to view ethnographies, phenomenologies, grounded theories, and the like as writing practices that themselves required study and even resistance, and to experiment with more artistic ways of representing Others and more participatory ways of authorizing these Others to represent themselves. The crisis of representation continues to generate literature emphasizing the literary, performative, and discursive aspects of inquiry and research dissemination (e.g., Cheek, 1996; Clifford & Marcus, 1986; Denzin & Lincoln, 2005; Geertz, 1988; Richardson, 2000; Tierney, 1995; Van Maanen, 1988; Wolf, 1992).

As we have often noted throughout this book, the research report, or the material form in which ethnographies, grounded theories, and the like are most often disseminated, is conventionally viewed as a reflection of what took place in a study. The research report is thought to reprise the study but not to be a component or shaper of it; it is typically conceived as a copy of an event, not an event itself. Yet scholars in such fields as cultural, gender, and social science and technology studies have increasingly troubled the notion that entities such as the medical record, the cardiac rhythm strip, the anatomy book, and the research report merely reflect reality (e.g., Berg, 1996; Latour & Woolgar, 1986; Lynch & Edgerton, 1988; Waldby, 2000). They have argued that these representations produce reality and, in fact, constitute the reality apprehended as the patient (in the record and rhythm strip), the body (in the anatomy book), and the study (in the report), respectively. The research report does not mirror a study but rather plays an active role in producing what is conventionally understood to be a study. The research report constitutes a writing practice that shapes what comes to be taken as scientific knowing and knowledge as studies are written up to conform to prescribed forms for reporting research, most notably, the APA/experimental style report (Bazerman, 1988).

Like research reports, which are traditionally viewed as reflections of what took place in a study, research findings are viewed as reflections of what took place in the lives of the research subjects who participated in that study. The qualitative research synthesis is thus viewed as a reflection of the findings across studies. Yet, as we have shown throughout this book, any synthesis of research findings is inevitably the result of a series of reviewer judgments (e.g., what questions to ask, what reports to include, what findings to feature) and of many rounds of transformations of information taken from research reports. Qualitative research syntheses are reviewers' constructions of researchers' constructions of the data that researchers generated in interaction with research participants, who constructed themselves and the events in their lives within the research encounter. The best access any inquirer can have in any context to someone else's experience-as-lived is via experience-as-told; qualitative research syntheses are, therefore, unavoidably far removed from the lived experiences they are meant faithfully to represent. The research syntheses that constitute the findings in reports of qualitative research synthesis studies can, thus, be read as if they were reasonably accurate reflections or copies of experience: as empirically grounded (albeit experientially-distant) interpretations of the lived experiences of the people who participated in the studies reviewed. Alternatively, in a more deconstructive vein, they can be read as narratives or discourses that reveal more about the research enterprise, the selves of the researchers who wrote the reports, and the selves of the reviewers who read them, than about the target experiences they were meant to feature.

Taking an Empirical/Analytical View

For example, we took an empirical/analytical view of research reports and findings to write up our qualitative metasynthesis of motherhood in HIV-positive women (Sandelowski & Barroso, 2003). We treated findings as if they were indexes of the experiences-as-lived of the women who participated in the studies reviewed and wrote them up to conform to the APA/experimental style of reporting empirical research. Indeed, the reports included in the Metasynthesis Project reflected a largely empirical/analytical "take." Among the integrated findings we reported were the following:

- Motherhood in the context of maternal HIV infection entailed work directed toward the illness itself and the social consequences of having HIV infection in the service of two primary goals: (a) the protection of children from HIV infection and HIV-related stigma and (b) the preservation of a positive maternal identity.
- Motherhood both intensified and mitigated the negative physical and social effects of HIV infection, while HIV infection, in turn, both interfered with and improved motherhood.
- The duality of motherhood in the context of maternal HIV infection appeared to reside not only in the paradoxical effects of motherhood and HIV infection on each other, but also in the contradictory effects of the same maternal action, and the common effects of contradictory actions.
- To counter the mortal and social threats of HIV infection and the contradictions of Western motherhood embodied in being an HIV-positive mother, the HIV-positive mothers studied variously

engaged in a distinctive kind of maternal practice aimed at both the preservation of children's lives and self-preservation as good mothers: virtual motherhood. Virtual motherhood signifies a maternal practice aimed at the preservation of children's lives and self-preservation as good mothers.

When we took an empirical/analytical view, we were operating (as we noted in chapter 8) "as if truth holds still" (Thorne, Jensen, Kearney, Noblit, & Sandelowski, 2004, p. 1354). Indeed, for qualitative metasynthesis to mean anything in the practice disciplines that emphasize usable knowledge, reviewers have to maintain truth as a "regulative ideal" (Murphy & Dingwall, 2001, p. 346): to sustain a primary commitment to producing "faithful accounts of a 'real' world," if not to big TRUTH, then to a "small(er)-'t' truth" (Michalowski, 1997, p. 67, n.1). This means assuming a stance of soft or "subtle realism" (Murphy & Dingwall, 2001, p. 346), accepting that "truths" outside of ourselves exist, even if they are inescapably socially constructed.

Taking a Critical/Discursive View

We then took a more critical/discursive view of these findings. Whereas the focus in our empirical reading of research reports with findings on motherhood in the context of HIV infection was on the actual experience of motherhood we took to be reflected in those findings (or "t-truths"), the focus in the discursive reading was on the talk of motherhood and what it accomplished. A discursive reading takes what is presented as research findings, not as empirically verifiable results generated from formal modes of data collection and analysis, but rather as the results of language and other social practices (i.e., discourses) involving researchers, research participants, and reviewers of research reports. Research findings are viewed, not as databased truths, but rather as historically and culturally contingent social products of unique encounters between reviewers and texts. These texts, in turn, are viewed as contingent products of an equally irreplicable and inescapably social interaction among multiple participant and researcher selves (Collins, 1998). Competing with a conventionally data-oriented view of research participants as informants or reporters are views of them as, for example, identity and impression managers, narrative strategists, and producers and objects of discourse (Grue & Laerum, 2002; Riessman, 1990; Sandelowski, 2002). Competing with the typical view of interview data as reasonably authentic accounts of facts and feelings is the view of them as, for example, public or private accounts (West, 1990), or as contributing to a "technology of biographical construction" (Atkinson & Silverman,

1997, p. 306). Competing with the data-oriented view of researchers and reviewers as reporters and integrators of findings are views of them as, for example, members of narrative or discourse communities, purveying collective stories, disciplinary values, methodological norms, and political agendas (Thorne et al., 2002).

Accordingly, taking a discursive view, we discerned in the reports we reviewed researchers' desire to offset negative images of HIV-positive women and to give voice to women they viewed as voiceless. As motherhood is arguably integral to the identity of every woman (whether or not she is or desires to be a mother; McMahon, 1996), talking about motherhood can be seen as a vehicle of communication for women that can cross any race, class, or other dividing line that might impede communication among them. The research participants in the HIV studies were women in largely marginalized social positions; the researchers were mostly women (who were, in turn, mostly nurses) in mainstream positions. The women participants wanted to offset negative images of HIV-positive women and to present themselves in a positive light. Indeed, the importance of motherhood to these women was not solely attributable to its importance to the researchers whose purpose was to study motherhood. Of the 56 qualitative reports of HIV-positive women with motherhood findings, 33 of them did not have as their research purpose to study motherhood at all. The women who participated in these studies themselves made motherhood salient, protesting the "spoiled identities" (Goffman, 1963) that emphasized their HIV status over their status as mothers. The caregiving professionals conducting these studies also wanted to offset the negative stereotypes of HIV-positive women and to present themselves as good listeners and compassionate interpreters. As a whole, the HIV reports reflected these researchers' view of HIV-positive women as "underdogs" requiring championing, and of qualitative research as founded upon the "metaphysics of the underdog" (Gouldner, 1968, p. 104; Jensen & Lauritsen, 2005, p. 63). As women and nurses too, we, in turn, wanted to present ourselves as competent interpreters and also to produce a research synthesis that would not contribute to the further stigmatization (or underdog status) of HIV-positive women. Motherhood talk allowed us all, in part, to achieve our goals (Grue & Laerum, 2002).

All of our talk here and elsewhere in this book about representation is to serve as a critical caveat to you: to alert you to the different takes (Cheek, 1996) on research reports available to you that will shape your write-up. Discursive readings of research reports can serve as an important corrective to claims reviewers make about experience-as-lived from empirical/analytical readings. Although offering a host of interpretations may seem at odds with the evidence-based practice imperative to offer one (albeit provisional) research synthesis, such methodological shape shifting optimizes the validity of research syntheses by virtue of acknowledging the disciplinary commitments and ideologies contributing to them. Critical readings serve as context, and even as alternative explanations, for the empirical/analytical readings constituting evidence syntheses. By offering alternative readings of the findings in research reports, qualitative research synthesis takes its place alongside quantitative meta-analysis in the evidence-based practice arena, but does not become so imitative of it that the critical imperatives of qualitative research are undermined (Barbour & Barbour, 2003; Sandelowski, 2006).

Reviewers can, like we did in Sandelowski and Barroso (2003), take an empirical/analytical view in one report, alluding to alternative view(s) in the discussion section. Reviewers can then use other reports to develop readings alternative to empirical/analytical ones, as exemplified in the research program of Barbara Paterson, Sally Thorne, and their colleagues (e.g., Paterson, Canam, Joachim, & Thorne, 2003; Thorne, Joachim, Paterson, & Canam, 2002; Thorne & Paterson, 1998; Thorne et al., 2002). Critical readings of research reports are not metasyntheses themselves (see chapter 2), but rather serve as foreground or background to empirical/analytical readings.

This tacking back and forth between different readings satisfies the agenda to "postmodernize" inquiry by adopting reflexive accounting practices (see chapter 8) and developing a sufficient amount of "representational humility" (Thorne et al., 2004, pp. 1352–1353). Reviewers acknowledge the language and social practices that constitute research reports and findings, while maintaining "t-truth" as a regulative ideal. As we previously noted, reviewers maintain contact with the empirical world as represented in research reports, while demonstrating their consciousness of research reports as literary technologies and of the interpretive acts and discursive practices entailed in any effort to synthesize research findings from reports (Alvesson & Sköldberg, 2000). The recognition of the crisis of representation posed by the qualitative research synthesis enterprise—of the representational issues in qualitative research synthesis and of qualitative research synthesis as itself constituting representation—will optimize the credibility and utility of the syntheses produced (Sandelowski, 2006).

THE ELEMENTS OF A REPORT OF A QUALITATIVE RESEARCH SYNTHESIS STUDY

Most journals publishing research syntheses will likely require that they be disseminated in the APA/experimental format, or a close variation of it. Accordingly, Table 9.1 summarizes and orders the contents that should appear in such write-ups of qualitative research synthesis studies. Because of the space restrictions in most journals, you will likely not be allowed to include all of the details of your method and all of the data available to support your synthesis. We found that different journals include and exclude different elements; for example, some journals did not allow us to include a citation list of all the primary research reports we reviewed or much detail on the thinking process behind the method choices we made. To offset this, many journals now have web sites to house such information. Moreover, you can indicate in your report what additional information is available to readers on request.

The irony here is that qualitative researchers, especially, are often blamed for not sufficiently articulating method, yet also continue to be charged with being too wordy or long-winded when they attempt to delineate method. The credibility of any research synthesis is undermined when reviewers are compelled to delete accounts of the key judgments that shaped their findings. In the research synthesis enterprise, objectivity resides in, and is an achievement of, such reflexive accounting practices. But the typical APA/experimental style report reflects and reproduces realist assumptions concerning inquiry and, thereby, does not accommodate well other inquiry positions. We have emphasized throughout this book that form is inseparable from and severely constrains content. How and what any one publication venue permits you to write will determine how and what you can write. These publication practices shape what comes to be accepted as knowledge. Indeed, Eisner (1997, p. 5) noted the "intimate relationship between our conception of what the products of research are to look like and the way we go about doing research."

FORMING THE SYNTHESIS

The heart of a report of a qualitative research synthesis study is the synthesis itself. You have several options here, even within the constraints of an experimental-style report. The one or more options you choose will depend on what the peculiarities of the data you are working with allow in the way of interpretation and representation, and on the audiences to which you want to appeal. "Appealing" reports are "convincing" texts that meet reader expectations (Golden-Biddle & Locke, 1993). For example, as illustrated in Tables 9.2 and 9.3, you may decide that a summary of meta-findings and their relative effect sizes produced from qualitative metasummary techniques, with each finding accompanied by a translation for practice, is most suitable for a largely clinical audience. (Another way of tabulating meta-summaries and effect sizes is shown in Table 6.3 in chapter 6.) Or, you may decide that a conceptual model or set of working hypotheses derived from a taxonomic analysis and/or reciprocal translation of concepts is most suitable for a largely research audience. Figures 9.1, 9.2, 9.3, and 9.4 show three conceptual renderings and one pictorial rendering of integrated findings. You will note that Figure 9.2 is a schematic version of the finding:

> Motherhood both intensified and mitigated the negative physical and social effects of HIV infection, while HIV infection, in turn, both interfered with and improved motherhood.

Figures 9.2 and 9.3 are schematic versions of the finding:

> The duality of motherhood in the context of maternal HIV infection appeared to reside not only in the paradoxical effects of motherhood and HIV infection on each other, but also in the contradictory effects of the same maternal action, and the common effects of contradictory actions.

Visual Displays

No matter what overall format you select, visual displays (e.g., graphs, charts, tables, lists, figures, schematic representations) will be useful to summarize volumes of information (as shown in Figure 9.1, Tables 9.2 and 9.3, and the tables shown in chapters 6 and 7), or to communicate a single idea involving disparate pieces of information (as shown in Table 9.4, and Figures 9.2 through 9.4). Key components of the "iconography of science" (Shapin, 1984, p. 491), visual displays function not only "manifestly" to reduce large quantities of data into forms that can be more readily apprehended by readers, but also "latently" to persuade readers of the validity of findings (McGill, 1990, p. 141). Because they are powerful rhetorical devices, you should spend as much time acquiring skills (or consulting with experts who have them) to create visual displays as you do in writing narrative text. The idea is to have displays that arrange information in ways that allow readers to see the comparisons you have made and the relationships you discerned. The only limits to your options are your imagination and what the publication venue you have chosen will allow.

Visual displays involve a decision on your part to organize information in certain ways. With the advent of computer media that emphasize the visual, excellent resources are being created every day to assist you to make good decisions concerning the visual displays of information in your study. Among these resources are Edward Tufte's *Envisioning Information* (1990) and *Visual Explanations* (1997), Harris' *Information Graphics* (1999), and Nicol's and Pexman's *Displaying Your Findings* (2003). For example, you will have to decide whether to construct matrices (rows and columns), networks (nodes and links), or Venn diagrams

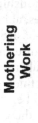

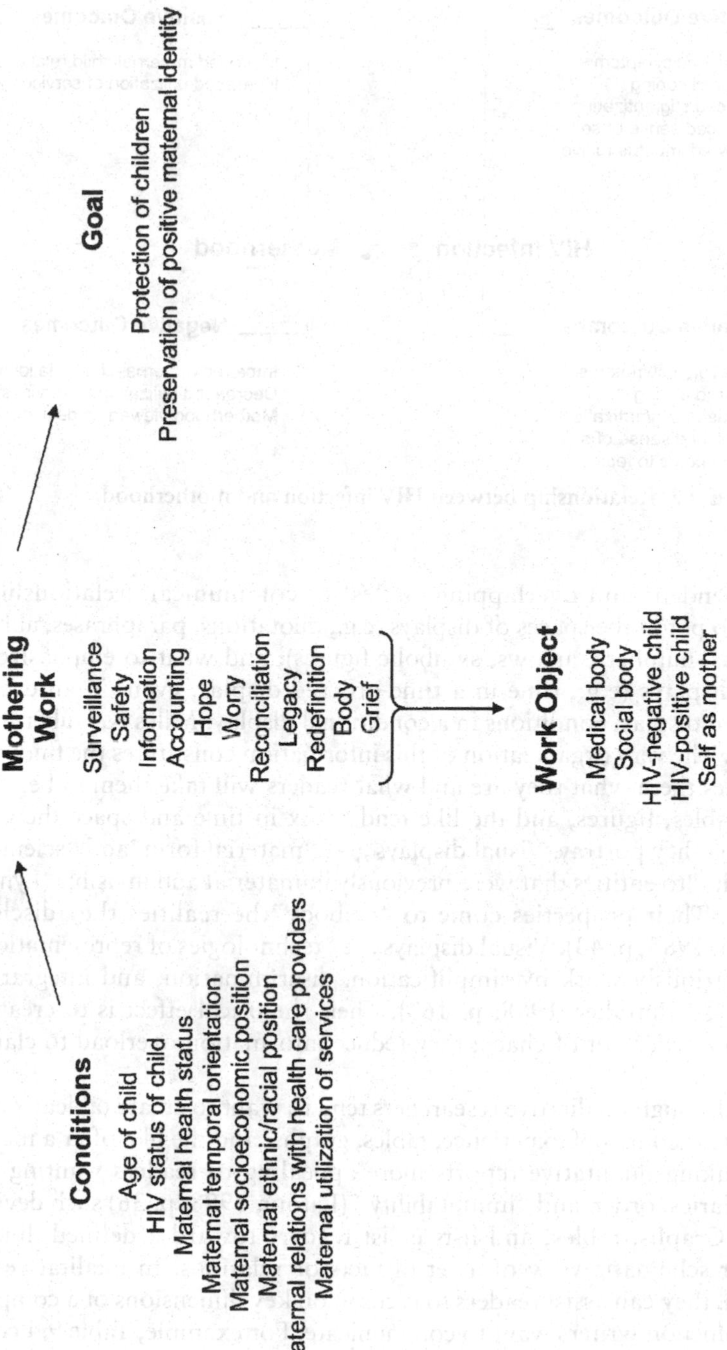

Goal

Protection of children
Preservation of positive maternal identity

Mothering Work

Surveillance
Safety
Information
Accounting
Hope
Worry
Reconciliation
Legacy
Redefinition
Body
Grief

Work Object

Medical body
Social body
HIV-negative child
HIV-positive child
Self as mother

Conditions

Age of child
HIV status of child
Maternal health status
Maternal temporal orientation
Maternal socioeconomic position
Maternal ethnic/racial position
Maternal relations with health care providers
Maternal utilization of services

FIGURE 9.1 Conceptual mapping of findings.

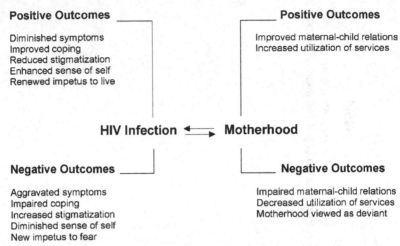

Positive Outcomes

Diminished symptoms
Improved coping
Reduced stigmatization
Enhanced sense of self
Renewed impetus to live

Positive Outcomes

Improved maternal-child relations
Increased utilization of services

HIV Infection ⟷ Motherhood

Negative Outcomes

Aggravated symptoms
Impaired coping
Increased stigmatization
Diminished sense of self
New impetus to fear

Negative Outcomes

Impaired maternal-child relations
Decreased utilization of services
Motherhood viewed as deviant

FIGURE 9.2 Relationship between HIV infection and motherhood.

(independent and overlapping circles) to communicate relationships; what to put in the spaces of displays (e.g., quotations, paraphrases, abbreviations, numbers, arrows, symbolic figures); and what to emphasize in your displays (e.g., time in a time-ordered display, event in an event-ordered display, conditions in a conditional display; Miles & Huberman, 1994). The very organization of this information constitutes the findings; it makes them what they are and what readers will take them to be.

Tables, figures, and the like tend to fix in time and space the phenomena they portray. Visual displays give "material form" and "scientific visibility" to entities that were previously immaterial and invisible (Lynch, 1985). Their properties come to "embody" the realities they disclose (Lynch, 1985, p. 43). Visual displays are "technologies of representation" that variously work by simplification, discrimination, and integration (Law & Whittaker, 1988, p. 163). Their rhetorical effect is to create a sense of order out of chaos; they reduce information overload to clarify meaning.

Although qualitative researchers tend to want to create tableaux and graphic accounts of experience, tables, graphs, and the like offer a means for making qualitative reports more appealing to readers wanting the boundaries, order, and "immutability" (Latour, 1988, p. 36) such devices offer. Graphs, tables, and lists enlist readers toward a defined, linear, and/or schematic view of a set of facts or relations. In qualitative research, they can assist readers to focus in on key dimensions of a complex phenomenon writers want to communicate. For example, Table 9.4 communicates how two opposing actions—disclosure and concealment—can

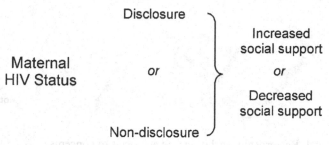

FIGURE 9.3 Contradictory relations.

lead to the same outcome (e.g., loss of social support) and how one action—disclosure—can lead to two opposing outcomes. Because such displays convey a "sense of proximity to the data collected" by the writer (McGill, 1990, p. 130), they tend to close the large gap that exists in any research synthesis project between research participants and reviewers of reports, and they lend support to the procedural rigor and interpretive credibility of the integrations produced.

Numbers

Numbers have been something of a "litmus test" (Linnekin, 1987, p. 920) of inquiry, serving in part to differentiate scientifically oriented/quantitative from humanistically oriented/qualitative research (Chibnik, 1999). Indeed, qualitative research is too often defined solely (and erroneously) by the absence and/or critique of numbers, whereas quantitative research is too often defined solely (and also erroneously) by the presence of numbers.

   Whether they appear in quantitative or qualitative research reports, numbers give studies rhetorical power by virtue of their association with science and objectivity. John (1992) proposed that statistics are a naturalized and rule-governed means of producing what is perceived to be the most conclusive knowledge about a target phenomenon. Statistics authorize studies as scientific and contribute to the "fixation of belief" whereby readers accept findings as facts and not as artifacts (Amann & Knorr-Cetina, 1988, p. 85). They are a display of evidence in the "artful literary display" (Gephart, 1988, p. 63) more familiarly known as the scientific report, and they are a means to create meaning. Indeed, quantitative significance is arguably less found than created, as writers rhetorically enlist readers to accept their findings as significant (Gephart, 1986). Statistical meaning is not "inherent in numbers," but rather "accomplished by terms used to describe and interpret numbers" (Gephart, 1988, p. 60).

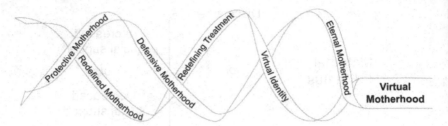

FIGURE 9.4 Reciprocal translation and synthesis of concepts.

In qualitative research, numbers have traditionally been looked upon with some suspicion as overly simplifying the complex. Indeed, qualitative researchers are often antagonistic to numbers, referring to their use as number-crunching and to those who use them as number-crunchers, and ranking numbers low in their "hierarchy of credibility" (Becker, 1967, p. 241). Qualitative researchers are especially concerned about the "dubious use" of numbers (Stern, 1989, p. 139) merely to authorize and legitimize qualitative work. Here writers become so preoccupied with providing exact numbers that they end up overcounting, or counting things that cannot or should not be counted. Overcounting will seriously detract from an aesthetic presentation of findings and, even more importantly, will divert attention away from the qualitative mandate to develop and present a fully rounded interpretation of things (Sandelowski, 2001).

Wanting to move "beyond numbers" (Greenhalgh & Taylor, 1997), qualitative researchers have often eschewed numbers as a violation of the imperatives of qualitative research. Numbers also present a representational problem to qualitative researchers who want to satisfy both scientific and humanistic/artistic criteria in their write-ups. Whereas quantitative researchers prize figures, qualitative researchers prize figures of speech. In short, although numbers are seen to confer epistemic authority in quantitative inquiry, they may also be seen to undermine the authority, authenticity, and artfulness of qualitative work.

Yet numbers are integral to qualitative analyses, especially for the recognition of patterns in data and deviations from those patterns, and for generalizing from data. Pattern recognition implies seeing something over and over again in one case or across a selection of cases. This repetition is the basis for qualitative metasummary. Finding that a *few, some,* or *many* reports showed a certain pattern, or that a pattern was *common* or *unusual* in a set of findings implies something about the frequency, typicality, or even intensity of an event. Anytime qualitative researchers place raw data into categories, or discover themes to which they attach codes, they are drawing from the numbered nature of phenomena for their analysis. Numbers are a powerful way to generate meaning from qualitative data; to document, verify, and test interpretations or conclusions; and to re-present target events and experiences.

Moreover, numbers are powerful devices to show the complexity and labor of qualitative work. Qualitative writers too often apologize for their "small" sample sizes, but do not show the large numbers of entities of which such ostensibly small samples are often actually comprised. In a qualitative research synthesis report, reviewers might convey, for example, the total pages of text comprising the primary data for their projects, and the numbers of participants and their characteristics represented across studies. In Barroso and Sandelowski (2003), we used several visual displays of numbers to communicate a summary profile of the women who participated in the HIV studies. In order to ascertain how well they represented the population of women with HIV infection, we compared (via tables and numbers) the women in these studies to women with HIV infection profiled in data from the Centers for Disease Control and Prevention (CDC). Because samples in research studies are often comprised solely of who is readily available to study, sample compositions may be neither statistically (ideal in quantitative research) nor informationally (ideal in qualitative research) representative. We wanted to determine the extent to which the women participating in these qualitative studies were representative of women known to have HIV disease and available to be included in national data sets such as those obtained by the CDC. This allowed us to situate the findings in these reports: that is, to evaluate what we knew about HIV-positive women by virtue of the women who participated in these studies and what we might still not know by virtue of the women who did not participate in them (Groger, Mayberry, & Straker, 1999).

Quotations

Although numbers tend to play a starring role in quantitative write-ups, quotations play a starring role in qualitative write-ups (Sandelowski, 1994). The quotation is arguably the analogue to the number, as they are both rhetorical devices used to appeal to readers to accept findings as scientifically and/or ethnographically valid. Quotations authenticate qualitative write-ups in that they demonstrate to readers that the writer has been "there," in the field (Geertz, 1988, Ch. 1), the closeness of the writer to the data and to the persons providing them (Richards, 1998), and the writer's attention to the "particulari(ties) of everyday life" (Golden-Biddle & Locke, 1993, p. 601). Whereas numbers are used in quantitative research write-ups primarily for their evidentiary power, quotations are used in qualitative research write-ups for their evidentiary power and their aesthetic value. Whereas numbers emphasize generality, quotations "privilege" individuality and "model . . . the diversity within generality" (Richardson, 1990, p. 40) that are hallmarks of qualitative research.

In qualitative research synthesis reports, reviewers quote researchers, not the participants researchers themselves quoted in their research reports. The primary data in qualitative research synthesis projects are the findings, or the researcher-generated interpretations of the data (including participant quotations) collected or generated in a primary study. Reviewers study the quotations researchers used to support their interpretations, but these quotations serve as evidence for researchers' interpretations (represented in the research findings), not for reviewers' syntheses of these findings. Quotations of researchers are used in write-ups of qualitative research synthesis projects to document reviewers' interpretations and to vitalize the presentation of reviewers' integration of findings. The functions of quoting in a qualitative research synthesis project is primarily to offer evidence for a reviewer conclusion or claim, to illustrate an interpretive point, and to represent the thinking of researchers about the persons and events they studied.

Like statistics and the work of statistics, quotations are rhetorical devices intended to persuade readers of the trustworthiness of a study, and quoting is a highly skilled craft that entails aesthetic and even moral choices. You must decide whether to quote at all; authenticity may be at stake if there are no quotations. You must then decide what, how, when, where, and why to quote. Such decisions include what segments of talk to quote, how to edit them, how to stage (that is, introduce and leave) them, where to use them (e.g., interspersed throughout the text, in sets in confined sections of the text, or in tabular displays), and why to use them (e.g., to convey the informational content or to evoke the feeling tone of an experience).

INNOVATIONS IN DISSEMINATION

You may also want to experiment with computer-mediated and artistic modalities for presenting your findings. We describe two such experiments here that we hope will serve as prototypes of and stimuli for other innovations in dissemination.

Disseminating Evidence Syntheses Via Digital Library

An innovation exploiting the appeal of computerized visual displays is the digital library we developed to disseminate the evidence syntheses we produced from qualitative findings pertaining to motherhood and stigma in

HIV-positive women. To design and evaluate this library, we followed a user-centered development approach (Fox et al., 1993). The entire development process is presented in Barroso, Edlin, Sandelowski, and Lambe (2006).

We turned to the digital library format to promote the accessibility of research findings to clinicians and, thereby, to enhance the utilization value of these findings. Despite the turn to evidence-based practice as a guiding principle and method in health care, too many of the findings from primary research studies have yet to make their way into practice. A persistent barrier to the use of research findings is the inaccessibility of research reports (Funk, Tornquist, & Champagne, 1995; Retsas, 2000). Researchers too often present their studies in ways that are incomprehensible and irrelevant to practitioners, and they may lack the presentation or translation skills to communicate findings in ways that are relevant to practice and provoke action. Practitioners, in turn, often do not have sufficient time, or the scientific literacy, numeracy, or methodological skills to read research or to conduct research synthesis projects. As we have emphasized throughout this book, research synthesis studies require skills, not only in understanding and evaluating the findings in individual research reports, but also in using advanced methods and techniques to synthesize the findings from multiple reports. They also require considerable information resources and expenditures of time that most health care professionals generally do not have. The SandBar Digital Library is an attempt to facilitate the transfer and use of information by offering an already integrated set of qualitative research findings in areas of practice especially relevant to improving the quality of life for HIV-positive women.

Digital libraries are extensions and augmentations of physical libraries (Marchionini & Fox, 1999). They combine the missions, techniques, and cultures of physical libraries with the capabilities and cultures of computing and telecommunications. Borgman (2000, p. 415) defined a digital library as:

> a system that provides a community of users with coherent access to a large, organized repository of information and knowledge . . . Digital libraries are a set of electronic resources and associated technological capabilities for creating, searching, and using information . . . They are constructed, collected, and organized by and for a community of users, and their functional capabilities support the information needs and uses of that community.

Digital libraries are extensions and enhancements of information retrieval systems. Among the distinguishing features of digital libraries are site neutrality, open access, greater variety and granularity of information, sharing of information, up-to-date–ness, continuous availability, and new forms of rendering information. The end result is that digital libraries shorten the chain from the author to the reader. This method of information distribution contributes to the concept of a collaboratory: a laboratory for geographically dispersed collaborators. Digital libraries accentuate the importance and increase the coverage of gray literature, an important but often difficult to retrieve component of comprehensive systematic reviews of research. Because people who use digital libraries have unique needs, another type of valuable service is personalization (Fox & Uhrs, 2002).

The SandBar Digital Library we created serves as a gateway to qualitative research findings on motherhood and stigma in HIV-positive women. Within each of these two major categories of research syntheses can be found the abstracted findings from the individual reports of studies, the effect size of each of the findings, and all reports containing similar findings. Citations can be searched by author name, title keyword, sample ethnicity, and/or year of publication. The Library also offers descriptions of the methods by which the findings were analyzed and synthesized. This Library closely resembles what Bishop (1999) described as the disaggregation and reaggregation of scientific and technical journal articles by students and faculty members. We rearranged and combined the critical elements of reports of studies to make them searchable and useful for clinicians and researchers working with HIV-positive women.

We invite you now to visit the SandBar Digital Library at http://sonweb.unc.edu/sandbar. To optimize its dissemination to key audiences, it is also housed at the web sites of the Well Project at http://www.thewell-project.org/index.jsp, and of the Association of Nurses in AIDS Care at http://www.anacnet.org/whatsnew.php.

Transforming an Evidence Synthesis Into Script and Video

An innovation embodying the growing interest of qualitative researchers in artistic modes of presenting research findings is the video we produced to represent them. Concurrent with the rise of evidence-based practice and its emphasis on research-based practice has been the increasing use of alternative modes of presenting qualitative research, or re-presenting the people and events that were its focus (Norris, 1997). Qualitative researchers have increasingly turned to forms of representation commonly associated with the humanities and arts in response to the (a) perceived "crisis of representation" (Smith, 2004, pp. 962–963) in qualitative research and the inadequacies of the traditional scientific research report faithfully and fairly to represent the lives of research participants, (b) growing rapprochement between the methods and imperatives of the social sciences and humanities, (c) desire to evoke more feeling (as opposed to purely cognitive) understandings (Van Manen, 1997) of human experience, and (d) desire to provoke action for social change rather than simply to report results. Qualitative researchers have transformed their research results into novels, poems, plays, dance, and other textual and performative forms completely out of the realm of scientific dissemination (see, e.g., Richardson's [2000] review of these forms and the journal, *Qualitative Inquiry*, which often features these forms). Although the turn to artistic modes of disseminating research findings is controversial in the qualitative research community (see, e.g., Sandelowski, 2004; Schwalbe, 1995), they offer ways to present research that may have more impact with audiences than the traditional research report.

The idea for creating a video to present a research synthesis came from an expert panel composed of nurses, social workers, and program administrators whose primary role was caring for persons with HIV infection. They participated in a series of focus groups concerning how best to move qualitative research findings into practice for a study we conducted that was directed toward this purpose.[1] After agreeing that stigma was a priority topic in their care of HIV-positive patients and subsequently reviewing the research syntheses in the forms shown in Tables 9.5 and Box 7.2 in chapter 7, the members of this expert panel recommended that a video be produced for HIV-positive women that they could view while waiting for their clinic appointments.

Accordingly, we collaborated with Frank Trimble, Chair of the Communications Studies Department at the University of North Carolina at Wilmington, who wrote the script to be faithful to the research findings and to satisfy the aesthetic requirements of script writing. He subsequently supervised its transformation into a 45-minute video entitled *HIV-Related Stigma in Five Voices*. Women viewers may choose to sit through the entire video, or select the segment featuring the (African American, Hispanic, or White) woman with whom they most identify.

The process we used to transform a research synthesis into script and video is fully described, and the entire script is shown, in Sandelowski, Trimble, Woodard, & Barroso (in press). If you are interested in obtaining the video, you may contact Frank Trimble.

AFTER SYNTHESIZING QUALITATIVE RESEARCH

After you have published the results of your synthesis project, you will have to decide whether you will continue to update your findings by beginning the synthesis process again with the additional studies completed after you closed your search. The results of your project may also have generated additional research questions that will motivate you to launch a program of research. No matter what your next step, your project will have contributed to developing the knowledge base for practice and to directing future research efforts and, thereby, to increasing the utilization value of qualitative research. You will also have gained a more finely honed appreciation for the complexity of research synthesis, in general, and qualitative research synthesis, in particular.

FINAL WORDS

We are pleased you chose to read our *Handbook* and hope it continues to help you in your efforts to synthesize qualitative research. We wish you well!

NOTE

1. This study was funded by a grant awarded to Betty Woodard (principal investigator) and us (coinvestigators) from the University of North Carolina at Chapel Hill School of Nursing Center for Research on Preventing and Managing Chronic Illness in Vulnerable Populations. This Center was funded by the National Institute of Nursing Research, National Institutes of Health (P30 NR03962, J. Harrell, Director, August 1, 1994–July 31, 2004).

TABLE 9.1 Template for Disseminating the Findings of Qualitative Research Synthesis Projects

1. Introduction
   a. Research problem that generated the study
   b. Research purpose addressing the research problem
2. Methods
   a. Sampling strategy
      i. Topical/thematic, population, temporal, & methodological boundaries
      ii. Key definitions and search terms
      iii. Inclusion & exclusion criteria
      iv. Channels of communication and information sources
      v. Goals of search strategy
      vi. Tools used to conduct searches & track search outcomes
   b. Techniques & tools used to appraise individual reports
   c. Techniques & tools used to compare reports
   d. Techniques & tools used to classify findings
   e. Methods, techniques, & tools used to synthesize findings
   f. Techniques & tools used to optimize the validity of study procedures
3. Results of review
   a. Sample configuration
      i. Profile of reports
         1. Number & findings type of primary research reports
         2. Inclusive years of reports
         3. Primary author disciplinary affiliation & nationality
         4. Geographic location of studies
         5. Purpose of studies
         6. Theoretical & methodological orientation of studies
         7. Relationship of reports (e.g., identical or overlapping samples)
         8. A posteriori analyses—e.g., by quality or other characteristic—of contributions of reports to synthesis
      ii. Profile of samples represented in reports
         1. Total and mean/median/modal sample size across reports
         2. Age, sex, racial/ethnic, class, national (& any other relevant demographic) composition of samples
         3. Other features of sample composition relevant to the purpose of the review and target phenomenon (e.g., stage of illness or pregnancy, diagnostic tests, treatment modalities)
   b. Synthesis of findings
      i. Narrative summary & delineation of key findings
      ii. Visual displays of findings
4. Discussion of findings (i.e., the synthesis produced)
   a. Link to existing scholarship
   b. Implications for research
   c. Implications for practice
   d. Limitations of the study
      i. Distinctive challenges to synthesis encountered
   e. Alternative to empirical/analytical reading of primary research findings (suggested here, and may be the focus of another paper)
5. List of complete citations to primary research reports (may be embedded in one end-of-text reference list with asterisks)
6. Acknowledgments, including grant support

TABLE 9.2 Illustration of Frequency Effect Size Table

Findings	Effect sizes (%)
1. A positive or suspicious prenatal diagnosis set into motion a series of nested and time-sensitive decisions, most notably: (a) whether to continue or terminate an affected pregnancy; and if terminating, (b) the mode of termination, (c) whether to view fetal remains, (d) how to handle fetal remains, and (e) whether and what to tell others (Alteneder et al., 1998; Bryar, 1997; Furlong & Black, 1984; Helm et al., 1998; Kolker et al., 1993; Menary, 1987; Oustifine, 1990; Rapp, 1988, 2000; Rillstone, 1999; Rillstone & Hutchinson, 2001; Rothman, 1986; Sandelowski & Jones, 1996a,b; Vantine, 2000).	100
2 Couples obtaining positive prenatal diagnoses managed information coming in to them pertaining to the diagnosis and the decisions they had to make by: (a) seeking information to make these decisions, affirm a decision already made, come to terms with the diagnosis, and learn about or verify the diagnosis; and (b) avoiding information that might undermine or cause them to regret a decision already made or acted on (Alteneder, 1998; Bryar, 1997; Furlong & Black, 1984; Helm et al., 1998; Matthews, 1990; Menary, 1987; Oustifine, 1990; Redlinger-Grosse et al., 2002; Rapp, 1988, 2000; Rillstone, 1999; Rillstone & Hutchinson, 2001; Rothman, 1986; Vantine, 2000).	80
3. Although difficult for men, positive prenatal diagnosis was devastating for women as it—and its aftermath— were embodied experiences for women (i.e., prenatal testing, quickening, the continuation or termination of a pregnancy with an impaired fetus, and postpartum leaking of breast milk happen in women's bodies) (Bryar, 1997; Furlong & Black, 1984; Kolker & Burke, 1993; Menary, 1987; Oustifine, 1990; Rapp, 1988, 2000; Rillstone, 1999; Rillstone & Hutchinson, 2001; Rothman, 1986; Vantine, 2000).	60

TABLE 9.3 Research Synthesis Shown as Meta-Findings With Clinical Translations

Meta-Finding

Couples obtaining positive prenatal diagnoses managed information coming in to them pertaining to the diagnosis and the decisions they had to make by: (a) seeking information to make these decisions, affirm a decision already made, come to terms with the diagnosis, and learn about or verify the diagnosis; and (b) avoiding information that might undermine or cause them to regret a decision already made or acted on (Alteneder et al., 1998; Bryar, 1997; Furlong & Black, 1984; Helm et al., 1998; Matthews, 1990; Menary, 1987; Oustifine, 1990; Rapp, 1988, 2000; Redlinger-Grosse et al., 2002; Rillstone, 1999; Rillstone & Hutchinson, 2001; Rothman, 1986; Vantine, 2000). In contrast, couples terminating pregnancies following positive prenatal diagnoses managed information going out from them pertaining to the decisions they had made by fully or partially disclosing to, or concealing the diagnosis and its aftermath from, children, other family members, friends, and acquaintances in order to obtain or preserve social support, protect them from the burden of knowledge, and avoid social condemnation (Bryar, 1997; Furlong & Black, 1984; Rapp, 1988, 2000; Vantine, 2000).

Clinical Translation

Clinicians must consider more than just the contents of information attending to couples' needs. *When* information is offered to couples is as important as *what* information is offered. Equally as relevant are the direction and goal of couples' information management efforts. For example, couples may be initially reluctant to see the remains or read reports of autopsies of their babies, but later decide they want this information. Couples sought to control information going out largely to minimize stigmatization, but they sought to control information coming in largely to reduce cognitive dissonance.

Meta-Finding

Positive prenatal diagnosis engendered an existential crisis in couples because it demanded that they choose the fate of their unborn child and, in the process, confront, reconcile, and subsequently act on their beliefs about human imperfection and disability, the obligations of parenthood, and the acceptability of abortion (Bryar, 1997; Menary, 1987; Rapp, 1988, 2000; Rothman, 1986; Sandelowski & Jones, 1996b; Vantine, 2000).

Clinical Translation

Clinicians should pay special attention to the particular constructions of choice couples receiving positive prenatal diagnoses use both to communicate and to come to terms with the event. This assessment of couples' narrative coping is key to assisting them to develop narrative strategies conducive to recovery and healing and to clinicians adopting a language that does not undermine these coping efforts. In narrative terms, clinicians' efforts to understand how couples "story" their encounter with positive diagnosis is a form of diagnosis. Intervention is then directed toward assisting couples to construct stories of choosing they can comfortably live with.

TABLE 9.4 Benefits and Risks of Disclosure and Concealment

	Benefits	Risks
Disclosure	Social support	Social isolation
	Access to health and social services	Diminished access to health and social services
		Discrimination in employment and housing
		Violence
	Sense of control and empowerment	Loss of control
	Improved self-image and self-healing	Damaged self-image
	Sense of pride and accomplishment	
	Relationship authenticity	
	Relief from secrecy and rumor	
Concealment	Social support	Social isolation
	Access to health and social services	Diminished access to health and social services
	Sense of control	Loss of control
	Maintenance of moral identity	Damaged self-image
	Privacy	Burden of secrecy and rumor
		Relationship inauthenticity
		Transmission of HIV infection

TABLE 9.5 Major Stigma Findings in Order of Prevalence

Women feared and experienced the negative social effects—on family and personal identity and authenticity—of disclosure, including social rejection, discrimination, and violence.

Women feared, anticipated, experienced, and adjusted their daily lives to the overt and covert stigmatization they attributed to their HIV infection in both close and distant relationships.

Disclosure of HIV was a major issue, dilemma, or stressor in women's lives.

Women internalized stigma, feeling shamed, blamed, guilt, worthless, dirty, deadly, deviant, and deficient as women and as mothers because they had HIV.

Factors influencing mothers' concerns and behavior regarding disclosure of their HIV to their children included the perceived inability of young children to understand or cope with the effects of maternal HIV, or to keep it a secret; the negative effects on children of HIV-related stigma; their own health and emotional state; the desire to protect their children; and the desire to preserve good relations with them.

Women described the positive effects of disclosure, including ease of further disclosure, healing, self-understanding, authenticity, empowerment, relief, support, sense of purpose, feelings of accomplishment and pride, and respite from secrets and rumors.

Of all the people to whom they might disclose, women were most or specifically concerned about disclosing their HIV to their children.

Women experienced discrimination in their interactions with health care providers, including mistreatment, indifference, providers not wanting to care for or touch them, comments implying that they deserved HIV, questions concerning how they contracted HIV, chart labels, lack of discretion, wearing multiple pairs of gloves, and pressure not to reproduce.

After disclosure, relationships remained close or distant, or became closer or more distant.

Being a woman, being a minority woman, being a mother, and being in or assumed to be in a stigmatizing circumstance other than HIV (e.g., drug use, prostitution, promiscuity, poverty, homelessness) had an additive effect on the stigma of HIV.

Women experienced keeping HIV a secret as a burden, requiring that they lead a double life, have only limited resources and relations, or lie.

Women engaged in considered, careful, or calculated disclosure of their HIV+ status, including determining when, what, and to whom to disclose.

Women assumed open, closed, and selective disclosure styles: i.e., telling everyone in their lives, telling everything, suppressing their diagnosis, disclosing immediately, delaying disclosure, deferring to others to disclose, passing, lying, and avoiding disclosure situations.

Women were ambivalent about disclosing their HIV to potential and actual male sex partners as partners' failure to disclose their own HIV was the reason for their infection and a cause of mistrust, and partners might reject them.

REFERENCES

Alvesson, M., & Sköldberg, K. (2000). *Reflexive methodology: New vistas for qualitative research*. London: Sage.

Amann, K., & Knorr-Cetina, K. (1988). The fixation of visual evidence. In M. Lynch & S. Woolgar (Eds.), *Representation in scientific practice* (pp. 85–121). New York: Kluwer Academic.

Atkinson, P., & Silverman, D. (1997). Kundera's immortality: The interview society and the invention of the self. *Qualitative Inquiry, 3*, 304–325.

Barbour, R. S., & Barbour, M. (2003). Evaluating and synthesizing qualitative research: The need to develop a distinctive approach. *Journal of Evaluation in Clinical Practice, 9*, 179–186.

Barroso, J., Edlin, A., Sandelowski, M., & Lambe, C. (2006). Bridging the gap between research and practice: The development of a digital library of research syntheses. *CIN: Computers, Informatics, Nursing, 24*, 85–94

Barroso, J., & Sandelowski, M. (2003). Sample reporting in qualitative studies of women with HIV infection. *Field Methods, 15*, 386–404.

Bazerman, C. (1988). *Shaping written knowledge: The genre and activity of the experimental article in science*. Madison: University of Wisconsin Press.

Becker, H. S. (1967). Whose side are we on? *Social Problems, 14*, 239–247.

Berg, M. (1996). Practices of reading and writing: The constitutive role of the patient record in medical work. *Sociology of Health & Illness, 18*, 499–524.

Bishop, A. P. (1999). Document structure and digital libraries: How researchers mobilize information in journal articles. *Information Processing & Management, 35*, 255–279.

Borgman, C. L. (2000). Digital libraries and the continuum of scholarly communications. *Journal of Documentation, 56*, 412–430.

Cheek, J. (1996). Taking a view: Qualitative research as representation. *Qualitative Health Research, 6*, 492–505.

Chibnik, M. (1999). Quantification and statistics in six anthropology journals. *Field Methods, 11*, 146–157.

Clifford, J., & Marcus, G. E. (Eds.). (1986). *Writing culture: The poetics and politics of ethnography*. Berkeley: University of California Press.

Collins, P. (1998). Negotiating selves: Reflections on unstructured interviewing. *Sociological Research Online, 3(3)*. Retrieved April 14, 2003, from http://www.socresonline.org.uk /3/3/2.html

Denzin, N. K., & Lincoln, Y. S. (2000). The discipline and practice of qualitative research. In N. K. Denzin & Y. S. Lincoln (Eds.), *Handbook of qualitative research* (2nd ed., pp. 1–28). Thousand Oaks, CA: Sage.

Denzin, N. K., & Lincoln, Y. S. (Eds.). (2005) *The Sage handbook of qualitative research* (3rd ed., pp. 165–181). Thousand Oaks, CA: Sage.

Eisner, E. W. (1997). The promise and perils of alternative forms of data representation. *Educational Researcher, 26 (6)*, 4–10.

Fox, E. A., Hix, D., Nowell, L. T., Brueni, D. J., Wake, W. C., et al. (1993). Users, user interfaces, and objects: Envision, a digital library. *Journal of the American Society for Information Science, 44*, 480–491.

Fox, E. A., & Urs, S. R. (2002). Digital libraries. In B. Cronin (Ed.), *Annual review of information science & technology* (Vol. 36, pp. 503–589). Medford: Information Today.

Funk, S. G., Tornquist, E. M., & Champagne, M. T. (1995). Barriers and facilitators of research utilization. *Nursing Clinics of North America, 30,* 395–407.

Geertz, C. (1988). *Works and lives: The anthropologist as author.* Stanford, CA: Stanford University Press.

Gephart, R. P. (1986). Deconstructing the defense for quantification in social science: A content analysis of journal articles on the parametric strategy. *Qualitative Sociology, 9,* 126–144.

Gephart, R. P. (1988). *Ethnostatistics: Qualitative foundations for quantitative research.* Beverly Hills, CA: Sage.

Goffman, E. (1963). *Stigma: Notes on the management of spoiled identity.* Englewood Cliffs, NJ: Prentice-Hall.

Golden-Biddle, K., & Locke, K. (1993). Appealing work: An investigation of how ethnographic texts convince. *Organization Science, 4,* 595–616.

Gouldner, A. (1968). The sociologist as partisan: Sociology and the welfare state. *American Sociologist, 3,* 103–116.

Greenhalgh, T., & Taylor, R. (1997). How to read a paper: Papers that go beyond numbers (qualitative research). *British Medical Journal, 315,* 740–743.

Groger, L., Mayberry, P. S., & Straker, J. K. (1999). What we didn't learn because of who would not talk to us. *Qualitative Health Research, 9,* 829–835.

Grue, L., & Laerum, K. T. (2002). "Doing motherhood": Some experiences of mothers with physical disabilities. *Disability & Society, 17,* 671–683.

Harris, R. L. (1999). *Information graphics: A comprehensive illustrated reference.* New York: Oxford University Press.

Jensen, C., & Lauritsen, P. (2005). Qualitative research as partial connection: Bypassing the power-knowledge nexus. *Qualitative Research, 5,* 59–77.

John, I. D. (1992). Statistics as rhetoric in psychology. *Australian Psychologist, 27,* 144–149.

Latour, B. (1988). Drawing things together. In M. Lynch & S. Woolgar (Eds.), *Representation in scientific practice* (pp. 19–68). New York: Kluwer Academic.

Latour, B., & Woolgar, S. (1986). *Laboratory life: The construction of scientific facts.* Princeton, NJ: Princeton University Press.

Law, J., & Whittaker, J. (1988). On the art of representation: Notes on the politics of visualization. In G. Fyfe & J. Law (Eds.), *Picturing power: Visual depiction and social relations* (pp. 160–183). London: Routledge.

Lincoln, Y. S., & Denzin, N. K. (2000). The seventh moment: Out of the past. In N. K. Denzin & Y. S. Lincoln (Eds.), *Handbook of qualitative research* (2nd ed., pp. 1047–1065). Thousand Oaks, CA: Sage.

Linnekin, J. (1987). Categorize, cannibalize? Humanistic quantification in anthropological research. *American Anthropologist, 89,* 920–926.

Lynch, M. (1985). Discipline and the material form of images: An analysis of scientific visibility. *Social Studies of Science, 15,* 37–66.

Lynch, M., & Edgerton, S. Y. (1988). Aesthetics and digital image processing: Representational craft in contemporary astronomy. In G. Fyfe & J. Law

(Eds.), *Picturing power: Visual depiction and social relations* (pp. 184–220). London: Routledge.

Marchionini, G., & Fox, E. (1999). Progress toward digital libraries: Augmentation through integration. *Information Processing & Management, 35,* 219–225.

McGill, L. T. (1990). Doing science by the numbers: The role of tables and other representational conventions in scientific journal articles. In A. Hunter (Ed.), *The rhetoric of social research: Understood and believed* (pp. 129–141). New Brunswick, NJ: Rutgers University Press.

McMahon, M. (1996). Significant absences. *Qualitative Inquiry, 2,* 320–336.

Michalowski, R. J. (1997). Ethnography and anxiety: Field work and reflexivity in the vortex of U.S.-Cuban relations. In R. Hertz (Ed.), *Reflexivity & voice* (pp. 45–69). Thousand Oaks, CA: Sage.

Miles, M. B., & Huberman, A. M. (1994). *Qualitative data analysis: An expanded sourcebook* (2nd ed.). Thousand Oaks, CA: Sage.

Murphy, E., & Dingwall, R. (2001). The ethics of ethnography. In P. Atkinson, A. Coffey, S. Delamont, J. Lofland, & L. Lofland (Eds.), *Handbook of ethnography* (pp. 339–351). London: Sage.

Nicol, A. A., & Pexman, P. N. (2003). *Displaying your findings: A practical guide for creating figures, posters, and presentations.* Washington, DC: American Psychological Association.

Norris, J. R. (1997). Meaning through form: Alternative modes of knowledge representation. In J. M. Morse (Ed.), *Completing a qualitative project: Details and dialogue* (pp. 87-115). Thousand Oaks, CA: Sage.

Paterson, B., Canam, C., Joachim, G., & Thorne, S. (2003). Embedded assumptions in qualitative studies of fatigue. *Western Journal of Nursing Research, 25,* 119–133.

Retsas, A. (2000). Barriers to using research evidence in nursing practice. *Journal of Advanced Nursing, 31,* 599–606.

Richards, L. (1998). Closeness to data: Goals of qualitative data handling. *Qualitative Health Research, 8,* 319–328.

Richardson, L. (1990). *Writing strategies: Reaching diverse audiences.* Newbury Park, CA: Sage.

Richardson, L. (2000). Writing: A method of inquiry. In N. K. Denzin & Y. S. Lincoln (Eds.), *Handbook of qualitative research* (2nd ed; pp. 923–948). Thousand Oaks, CA: Sage.

Riessman, C. K. (1990). Strategic uses of narrative in the presentation of self and illness: A research note. *Social Science & Medicine, 30,* 1195–1200.

Sandelowski, M. (1994). The use of quotes in qualitative research. *Research in Nursing & Health, 17,* 479–482.

Sandelowski, M. (2001). Real qualitative researchers do not count: The use of numbers in qualitative research. *Research in Nursing & Health, 24,* 230–240.

Sandelowski, M. (2002). Reembodying qualitative inquiry. *Qualitative Health Research, 12,* 104–115.

Sandelowski, M. (2004). Using qualitative research. *Qualitative Health Research, 14,* 1366–1386.

Sandelowski, M. (2006). "Meta-jeopardy": The crisis of representation in qualitative metasynthesis. *Nursing Outlook, 54,* 10–16.

Sandelowski, M., & Barroso, J. (2003). Motherhood in the context of maternal HIV infection. *Research in Nursing & Health, 26,* 470–482.

Sandelowski, M., Trimble, F., Woodard, E. K., & Barroso, J. (in press). From synthesis to script: Transforming qualitative research findings for use in practice. *Qualitative Health Research.*

Schwalbe, M. (1995). The responsibilities of sociological poets. *Qualitative Sociology, 18,* 393–413.

Shapin, S. (1984). Pump and circumstance: Robert Boyle's literary technology. *Social Studies of Science, 14,* 481–520.

Smith, J. K. (2004). Representation, crisis of. In M. S. Lewis-Beck, A. Bryman, & T. F. Liao (Eds.), *The Sage encyclopedia of social science research methods* (Vol. 3, pp. 962–963). Thousand Oaks, CA: Sage.

Stern, P. N. (1989). Are counting and coding a cappella appropriate in qualitative research? In J. M. Morse (Ed.), *Qualitative nursing research: A contemporary dialogue* (pp. 135–148). Rockville, MD: Aspen.

Thorne, S., Jensen, L., Kearney, M. H., Noblit, G., & Sandelowski, M. (2004). Qualitative metasynthesis: Reflections on methodological orientation and ideological agenda. *Qualitative Health Research, 14,* 1342–1365.

Thorne, S., Joachim, G., Paterson, B., Canam, C. (2002). Influence of the research frame on qualitatively derived health science. *International Journal of Qualitative Methods, 1(1).* Article 1. Retrieved March 14, 2003, from http://www.ualberta.ca/~ijqm/english/engframeset.html

Thorne, S., & Paterson, B. (1998). Shifting images of chronic illness. *Image: Journal of Nursing Scholarship, 30,* 173–178.

Thorne, S., Paterson, B., Acorn, A., Canam, C., Joachim, G., & Jillings, C. (2002). Chronic illness experience: Insights from a metastudy. *Qualitative Health Research, 12,* 437–452.

Tierney, W. G. (1995). (Re)Presentation and voice. *Qualitative Inquiry, 1,* 379–390.

Tufte, E. R. (1990). *Envisioning information.* Cheshire, CT: Graphics Press.

Tufte, E. R. (1997). *Visual explanations: Images and quantities, evidence and narrative.* Cheshire, CT: Graphics Press.

Van Maanen, J. (1988). *Tales of the field: On writing ethnography.* Chicago: University of Chicago Press.

Van Manen, M. (1997). From meaning to method. *Qualitative Health Research, 7,* 345–369.

Waldby, C. (2000). *The Visible Human Project: Informatic bodies and posthuman medicine.* New York: Routledge.

West, P. (1990). The status and validity of accounts obtained at interview: A contrast between two studies of families with a disabled child. *Social Science & Medicine, 30,* 1229–1239.

Wolf, M. (1992). *A thrice-told tale: Feminism, postmodernism, and ethnographic responsibility.* Stanford, CA: Stanford University Press.

APPENDIX

Reports in the Qualitative Metasynthesis Project

HIV Reports

Published Reports

Andrews, S., Williams, A. B., & Neil, K. (1993). The mother-child relationship in the HIV-1 positive family. *Image: Journal of Nursing Scholarship, 25*, 193–198.

Barnes, D. B., Taylor-Brown, S., & Wiener, L. (1997). "I didn't leave y'all on purpose": HIV-infected mothers' videotaped legacies for their children. *Qualitative Sociology, 20*, 7–32.

Bedimo, A. L., Bennett, M., Kissinger, P., & Clark, R. A. (1998). Understanding barriers to condom usage among HIV-infected African American women. *Journal of the Association of Nurses in AIDS Care, 9*, 48–58.

Black, B. P., & Miles, M. S. (2002). Calculating the risks and benefits of disclosure in African American women who have HIV. *JOGNN: Journal of Obstetric, Gynecologic, & Neonatal Nursing, 31*, 688–697.

Bunting, S. M., & Seaton, R. (1999). Health care participation of perinatal women with HIV: What helps and what gets in the way? *Health Care for Women International, 20*, 563–578.

Chin, D., & Kroesen, K. W. (1999). Disclosure of HIV infection among Asian/Pacific Islander American women: Cultural stigma and support. *Cultural Diversity and Ethnic Minority Psychology, 5*, 222–235.

Ciambrone, D. A. (2001). Illness and other assaults on self: The relative impact of HIV/AIDS on women's lives. *Sociology of Health & Illness, 23*, 517–540.

Ciambrone, D. A. (2002). Informal networks among women with HIV/AIDS: Present support and future prospects. *Qualitative Health Research, 12*, 876–896.

Coward, D. D. (1995). The lived experience of self-transcendence in women with AIDS. *JOGNN: Journal of Obstetric, Gynecologic and Neonatal Nursing, 24*, 314–318.

Crane, J. R., Perlman, S., Meredith, K. L., Jeffe, D. B., Fraser, V. J., Lucas, A. M., & Mundy, L. M. (2000). Women with HIV: Conflicts and synergy of prayer within the realm of medical care. *AIDS Education and Prevention*, 12, 532–543.

DeMarco, R. F., Miller, K. H., Patsdaughter, C. A., Chisholm, M., & Grindel, C. G. (1998). From silencing the self to action: Experiences of women living with HIV/AIDS. *Health Care for Women International*, 19, 539–552.

Demi, A., Moneyham, L., Sowell, R., & Cohen, L. (1997). Coping strategies used by HIV infected women. *Omega*, 35, 377–391.

Dunbar, H. T., Mueller, C. W., Medina, C., & Wolf, T. (1998). Psychological and spiritual growth in women living with HIV. *Social Work*, 43, 144–154.

Faithfull, J. (1997). HIV-positive and AIDS-infected women: Challenges and difficulties of mothering. *American Journal of Orthopsychiatry*, 67, 144–151.

Gielen, A. C., O'Campo, P., Faden, R. R., & Eke, A. (1997). Women's disclosure of HIV status: Experiences of mistreatment and violence in an urban setting. *Women and Health*, 25, 19–31.

Goggin, K., Catley, D., Brisco, S. T., Engelson, E. S., Rabkin, J. G., & Kotler, D. P. (2001). A female perspective on living with HIV. *Health & Social Work*, 26, 80–89.

Goicoechea-Balbona, A., Barnaby, C., Ellis, I., & Foxworth, V. (2000). AIDS: The development of a gender appropriate research intervention. *Social Work in Health Care*, 30, 19–37.

Gramling, L., Boyle, J. S., McCain, N., Ferrell, J., Hodnicki, D., & Muller, R. (1995). Reconstructing a woman's experiences with AIDS. *Family and Community Health*, 19, 49–56.

Gray, J. J. (1999). The difficulties of women living with HIV infection. *Journal of Psychosocial Nursing and Mental Health Services*, 37, 39–43.

Grove, K. A., Kelly, D. P., & Liu, J. (1997). "But nice girls don't get it": Women, symbolic capital, and the social construction of AIDS. *Journal of Contemporary Ethnography*, 26, 317–337.

Guillory, J. A., Sowell, R., Moneyham, L., & Seals, B. (1997). An exploration of the meaning and use of spirituality among women with HIV/AIDS. *Alternative Therapies in Health and Medicine*, 3, 55–60.

Hackl, K. L., Somlai, A. M., Kelly, J. A., & Kalichman, S. C. (1997). Women living with HIV/AIDS: The dual challenge of being a patient and caregiver. *Health and Social Work*, 22, 53–62.

Haile, B. L., Landrum, P. A., Kotarba, J. A., & Trimble, D. (2002). Inner strength among HIV infected women: Nurses can make a difference. *Journal of the Association of Nurses in AIDS Care*, 13, 74–80.

Hassin, J. (1994). Living a responsible life: The impact of AIDS on the social identity of intravenous drug users. *Social Science & Medicine*, 39, 391–400.

Hutchison, M., & Kurth, A. (1991). "I need to know that I have a choice": A study of women, HIV, and reproductive decision-making. *AIDS Patient Care*, 5, 17–25.

Ingram, D., & Hutchinson, S. A. (1999a). Defensive mothering in HIV-positive mothers. *Qualitative Health Research*, 9, 243–258.

Ingram, D., & Hutchinson, S. A. (1999b). HIV-positive mothers and stigma. *Health Care for Women International*, 20, 93–103.

Ingram, D., & Hutchinson, S. A. (2000). Double binds and the reproductive and mothering experiences of HIV-positive women. *Qualitative Health Research,* *10,* 117–132.

Kass, N., & Faden, R. (1996). In women's words: The values and lived experiences of HIV-infected women. In R. F. Faden & N. E. Kass (Eds.), *HIV, AIDS and childbearing: Public policy, private lives* (pp. 426–443). Oxford: Oxford University Press.

Kimberly, J. A., Serovich, J. M., & Greene, K. (1995). Disclosure of HIV-positive state: Five women's stories. *Family Relations, 44,* 316–322.

Lather, P., & Smithies, C. (1997). *Troubling the angels: Women living with HIV/AIDS.* Boulder, CO: Westview Press.

Leenerts, M. H. (1998). Barriers to self-care in a cohort of low-income White women living with HIV/AIDS. *Journal of the Association of Nurses in AIDS Care, 9,* 22–36.

Leenerts, M. H. (1999). The disconnected self: Consequences of abuse in a cohort of low-income white women living with HIV/AIDS. *Health Care for Women International, 20,* 381–400.

Leenerts, M. H., Flaskerud, J. H., & Saunders, J. (1999). Lingering images: Symbols and meanings of self-images in HIV-positive women with abuse histories. *National Academies of Practice Forum, 1,* 209–218.

Leenerts, M. H., & Magilvy, J. K. (2000). Investing in self-care: A midrange theory of self-care grounded in the lived experience of low-income HIV-positive white women. *Advances in Nursing Science, 22,* 58–75.

Litwak, E., Sudit, M., Baker, S., Dobkin, J., & Fullilove, M. (1995). *Caregiving needs of HIV-positive minority women.* Arlington, VA: United States Department of Commerce, National Technical Information Service.

Marcenko, M. O., & Samost, L. (1999). Living with HIV/AIDS: The voices of HIV-positive mothers. *Social Work, 44,* 36–45.

Misener, T. R., & Sowell, R. L. (1998). HIV-infected women's decisions to take antiretrovirals. *Western Journal of Nursing Research, 20,* 431–447.

Moneyham, L., Seals, B., Demi, A., Sowell, R., Cohen, L., & Guillory, J. (1996a). Experiences of disclosure in women infected with HIV. *Health Care for Women International, 17,* 209–221.

Moneyham, L., Seals, B., Demi, A., Sowell, R., Cohen, L., & Guillory, J. (1996b). Perceptions of stigma in women infected with HIV. *AIDS Patient Care and STDs, 10,* 162–167.

Morrow, K., Costello, T., & Boland, R. (2001). Understanding the psychosocial needs of HIV positive women: A qualitative study. *Psychosomatics, 42,* 497–503.

Moser, K. M., Sowell, R. L., & Phillips, K. D. (2001). Issues of women dually diagnosed with HIV infection and substance use problems in the Carolinas. *Issues in Mental Health Nursing, 22,* 23–49.

Murdaugh, C., Russell, R. B., & Sowell, R. (2000). Using focus groups to develop a culturally sensitive videotape intervention for HIV-positive women. *Journal of Advanced Nursing, 32,* 1507–1513.

Napravnik, S., Royce, R., Walter, E., & Lim, W. (2000). HIV-1 infected women and prenatal care utilization: Barriers and facilitators. *AIDS Patient Care and STDs, 14,* 411–420.

Raveis, V. H., Siegel, K., & Gorey, E. (1998). Factors associated with HIV-infected women's delay in seeking medical care. *AIDS Care, 10,* 549–562.

Regan-Kubinski, M. J., & Sharts-Hopko, N. (1995). Illness cognition of HIV-infected mothers. *Issues in Mental Health Nursing, 16,* 327–344.

Richter, D. L., Sowell, R. L., & Pluto, D. M. (2002). Attitudes toward antiretroviral therapy among African American women. *American Journal of Health Behavior, 26,* 25–33.

Rose, M. A. (1993). Health concerns of women with HIV/AIDS. *Journal of the Association of Nurses in AIDS Care, 4,* 39–45.

Russell, J. M., & Smith, K. V. (1999). A holistic life view of human immunodeficiency virus–infected African American women. *Journal of Holistic Nursing, 17,* 331–345.

Sankar, A., Luborsky, M., Schuman, P., & Roberts, G. (2002). Adherence discourse among African-American women taking HAART. *AIDS Care, 14,* 203–218.

Santacroce, S. J., Deatrick, J. A., & Ledlie, S. W. (2002). Redefining treatment: How biological mothers manage their children's treatment for perinatally acquired HIV. *AIDS Care, 14,* 247–260.

Schrimshaw, E. W., & Siegel, K. (2002). HIV-infected mothers' disclosure to their uninfected children: Rates, reasons, and reactions. *Journal of Social and Personal Relationships, 19,* 19–43.

Seals, B. F., Sowell, R. L., Demi, A. S., Moneyham, L., Cohen, L., & Guillory, J. (1995). Falling through the cracks: Social service concerns of women infected with HIV. *Qualitative Health Research, 5,* 496–515.

Semple, S. J., Patterson, T. L., Temoshok, L. R., McCutchan, J. A., Straits-Troster, K. A., Chandler, J. L., & Grant, I. (1993). Identification of psychobiological stressors among HIV-positive women. *Women and Health, 20,* 15–36.

Serovich, J. M., Kimberly, J. A., & Greene, K. (1998). Perceived family member reaction to women's disclosure of HIV-positive information. *Family Relations, 47,* 15–22.

Siegel, K., & Gorey, E. (1997). HIV-infected women: Barriers to AZT use. *Social Science & Medicine, 45,* 15–22.

Siegel, K., Lekas, H. M., Schrimshaw, E. W., & Johnson, J. K. (2001). Factors associated with HIV-infected women's use or intention to use AZT during pregnancy. *AIDS Education and Prevention, 13,* 189–206.

Siegel, K., Raveis, V. H., & Gorey, E. (1998). Barriers and pathways to testing among HIV-infected women. *AIDS Education and Prevention, 10,* 114–127.

Siegel, K., & Schrimshaw, E. W. (2000). Perceiving benefits in adversity: Stress-related growth in women living with HIV/AIDS. *Social Science & Medicine, 51,* 1543–1554.

Siegel K., & Schrimshaw, E. W. (2001). Reasons and justifications for considering pregnancy among women living with HIV/AIDS. *Psychology of Women Quarterly, 25,* 112–123.

Smith, K. V., & Russell, J. (1997). Ethical issues experienced by HIV-infected African-American women. *Nursing Ethics, 4,* 394–402.

Sowell, R. L., & Misener, T. R. (1997). Decisions to have a baby by HIV-infected women. *Western Journal of Nursing Research, 19,* 56–70.

Sowell, R. L., Moneyham, L., Guillory, J., Seals, B., Cohen, L., & Demi, A. (1997). Self-care activities of women infected with human immunodeficiency virus. *Holistic Nursing Practice, 11,* 18–26.

Sowell, R. L., Seals, B., Moneyham, L., Guillory, J., Demi, A., & Cohen, L. (1996). Barriers to health-seeking behaviors for women infected with HIV. *Nursing Connections, 9,* 5–17.

Stanley, L. D. (1999). Transforming AIDS: The moral management of stigmatized identity. *Anthropology and Medicine, 6,* 103–120.

Stevens, P. E. (1996). Struggles with symptoms: Women's narratives of managing HIV illness. *Journal of Holistic Nursing, 14,* 142–160.

Stevens, P. E., & Doerr, B. T. (1997). Trauma of discovery: Women's narratives of being informed they are HIV-infected. *AIDS Care, 9,* 523–538.

Stevens, P. E., & Richards, D. J. (1998). Narrative case analysis of HIV infection in a battered woman. *Health Care for Women International, 19,* 9–22.

Tangenberg, K. (2000). Marginalized epistemologies: A feminist approach to understanding the experiences of mothers with HIV. *Affilia, 15,* 31–48.

Tangenberg, K. M. (2001). Surviving two diseases: Addiction, recovery, and spirituality among mothers living with HIV disease. *Families in Society: The Journal of Contemporary Human Services, 82,* 517–524.

Tuchel, T. L., & Feldman, D. A. (1993). A preliminary ethnography of HIV-positive women in Dade County jails. *Practicing Anthropology, 15,* 52–55.

Valdez, M. D. (2001). A metaphor for HIV positive Mexican and Puerto Rican women. *Western Journal of Nursing Research, 23,* 517–535.

Van Loon, R. A. (2000). Redefining motherhood: Adaptation to role change for women with AIDS. *Families in Society: The Journal of Contemporary Human Services, 81,* 152–161.

Van Servellen, G., Sarna, L., & Jablonski, K. J. (1998). Women with HIV: Living with symptoms. *Western Journal of Nursing Research, 20,* 448–464.

Walker, S. E. (1998). *Women with AIDS and their children.* New York, NY: Garland Publishers.

Weitz, R. (1993). Powerlessness, invisibility, and the lives of women with HIV disease. *Advances in Medical Sociology, 3,* 101–121.

Wesley, Y., Smeltzer, S. C., Redeker, N., Walker, S., Palumbo, P., & Whipple, B. (2000). Reproductive decision making in mothers with HIV-1. *Health Care for Women International, 21,* 291–304.

Winstead, B. A., Derlega, V. J., Barbee, A. P., Sachdev, M., Antle, B., & Greene, K. (2002). Close relationships as sources of strength or obstacles for mothers coping with HIV. *Journal of Loss & Trauma, 7,* 157–184.

Woodard, B., & Sowell, R. L. (2001). God in control: Women's perspectives on managing HIV infection. *Clinical Nursing Research, 10,* 233–250.

Unpublished Reports

Armstrong, V. A. (1996). *The experience of the HIV-positive mother with an HIV-positive child: A descriptive study.* Unpublished doctoral dissertation, University of California at San Francisco.

Arnold, M. A. (1994). *Women with HIV disease: Psychosocial issues*. Unpublished doctoral dissertation, Massachusetts School of Professional Psychology, Boston.

Bell, E. M. (1997). *Women with AIDS: A qualitative study of their experiences and interactions with health care and its providers*. Unpublished doctoral dissertation, California School of Professional Psychology, Los Angeles.

Bennett, M. J. (1997). *Stigmatization experiences of HIV infected women: A focused ethnography*. Unpublished doctoral dissertation, Louisiana State University Medical Center, New Orleans.

Berger, M. T. (1998). *Workable sisterhood: A study of the political participation of stigmatized women with HIV/AIDS*. Unpublished doctoral dissertation, University of Michigan, Ann Arbor.

Bonifas, J. M. (1994). *The psychologic experience of women living with HIV/AIDS: A phenomenological study*. Unpublished doctoral dissertation, Union Institute, Union Graduate School, Cincinnati, OH.

Caba, G. (1998). *The struggle for meaning in the lives of HIV+ women*. Unpublished doctoral dissertation, University of Toledo, OH.

Cameron, A. E. (2001). *Narrative voice and countering silence: Women talk about life with AIDS*. Unpublished doctoral dissertation, City University of New York.

Ciambrone, D. A. (1999). *Mending fractured selves: Biographical disruption among women with HIV infection*. Unpublished doctoral dissertation, Brown University, Providence, RI.

Dominguez, L. M. (1996). *The lived experience of women of Mexican heritage with HIV/AIDS*. Unpublished doctoral dissertation, University of Arizona, Tucson.

Dozier, J. K. (1997). *Lived experience of HIV positive women*. Unpublished doctoral dissertation, Kent State University, Kent, OH.

Faithfull, J. (1992). *HIV, reproductive decision-making, and mothering experiences*. Unpublished Master's thesis, Smith College, Northampton, MA.

Frey, L. M. (1993). *The psychological and sociopolitical sequelae of HIV infection in women*. Unpublished doctoral dissertation, Antioch University, Keene, NH.

Gosling, A. (1995). *Pain, courage, and wisdom: Stories of women living with HIV*. Unpublished doctoral dissertation, Virginia Polytechnic Institute and State University, Blacksburg.

Hendrixson, L. L. (1996). *The psychosocial and psychosexual impact of HIV/AIDS disease on rural women: A qualitative study*. Unpublished doctoral dissertation, New York University, New York.

Ingram, D. A. (1996). *HIV-positive women: Double binds and defensive mothering*. Unpublished doctoral dissertation, University of Florida, Gainesville.

Knight, V. A. (1998). *The art of self-care: Self nurturance and the African-American women with HIV/AIDS*. Unpublished doctoral dissertation, Union Institute, Union Graduate School, Cincinnati, OH.

Leenerts, M. H. (1997). *Ways low-income white women manage life with HIV/AIDS*. Unpublished doctoral dissertation, University of Colorado Health Sciences Center, Denver.

Locher, A.W. (1995). *The lived experience of women who have perinatally infected their children with human immunodeficiency virus.* Unpublished Master's thesis, Medical College of Ohio, Toledo.

Loriz-Lim, L. M. (1995). *Women's explanations of living with HIV.* Unpublished doctoral dissertation, George Mason University, Fairfax, VA.

Noone, S. B. (2000). *Treading on thin ice: A qualitative study of women and HIV disclosure.* Unpublished doctoral dissertation, Union Institute, Union Graduate School, Cincinnati, OH.

Palyo, K. (1995). *Lived experience of women with HIV within a self-care framework.* Unpublished Master's thesis, Medical College of Ohio, Toledo.

Ritchie, M. G. (1996). *Psychosocial factors affecting healthcare utilization for women with HIV: A multiple clinical case study.* Unpublished doctoral dissertation, California Institute of Integral Studies, San Francisco.

Ross, T. L. (1994). *The lived experience of hope in young mothers with human immunodeficiency virus infection: A phenomenological inquiry.* Unpublished doctoral dissertation, Adelphi University, New York, NY.

Salmon, P. L. (1993). *Women's narratives: Living with HIV disease.* Unpublished doctoral dissertation, University of South Florida, Tampa.

Sepples, S. B. (1996). *Women's narratives of the experience of living with HIV infection.* Unpublished doctoral dissertation, University of Virginia, Charlottesville.

Tangenberg, K. M. (1998). *Marginalized epistemologies: Bodily and spiritual knowing among HIV-positive mothers.* Unpublished doctoral dissertation, University of Washington, Seattle.

Tanner, T. S. (1995). *Socialization and self-worth: An in-depth analysis of the effects of socialization as it relates to the lives of seven HIV positive women.* Unpublished Master's thesis, California State University, Dominguez Hills.

Valdez, M. D. (1999). *La Protectora (The Protectress): A metaphor for HIV+ Hispanic women.* Unpublished doctoral dissertation, Texas Woman's University, Denton.

Van Loon, R. A. (1996). *Coping and adaptation in women with AIDS.* Unpublished doctoral dissertation, University of Chicago, IL.

Walker, S. (1996). *Vertically transmitted HIV+/AIDS: The impact on maternal attachment.* Unpublished doctoral dissertation, Antioch University, Keene, NH.

Walsh, E. R. (2000). *Women's decision-making experiences regarding disclosure of HIV seropositivity: A qualitative study.* Unpublished doctoral dissertation, University of Michigan, Ann Arbor.

Williamson, M. (2000). *Life transformations of African-American HIV positive women: Possible implications for HIV policy making.* Unpublished doctoral dissertation, University of Chicago, IL.

Woodard, B. (2002). *How African American women in North Carolina use spirituality to manage HIV disease: A grounded theory.* Unpublished doctoral dissertation, University of South Carolina, Columbia.

Wright, E. M. (1995). *Deep from within the well: African-American women living with AIDS.* Unpublished doctoral dissertation, Syracuse University, NY.

HIV REPORTS WITH IDENTICAL OR SHARED SAMPLES

Identical Samples

Ciambrone, 1999, 2001, 2002
Faithfull, 1992, 1997
Leenerts, 1997, 1998, 1999; Leenerts & Magilvy, 2000; Leenerts, Flaskerud, &
    Saunders, 1999
Misener & Sowell, 1998; Sowell & Misener, 1997
Marcenko & Samost, 1999; Tangenberg, 1998, 2000, 2001
Moneyham et al., 1996a, b
Russell & Smith, 1999; Smith & Russell, 1997
Siegel, Lekas, Schrimshaw, & Johnson, 2001; Siegel & Schrimshaw, 2001
Stevens, 1996; Stevens & Doerr, 1997
Valdez, 1999, 2001
Van Loon, 1996, 2000

Overlapping or Shared Samples

Guillory, Sowell, Moneyham, Seals, 1997; Seals et al., 1995; Sowell et al., 1997;
    Sowell et al., , 1996
Ingram, 1996; Ingram & Hutchinson, 1999a, b, 2000
Kimberly, Serovich, & Greene, 1995; Serovich, Kimberly, & Greene, 1998
Raveis, Siegel, & Gorey, 1998; Siegel & Gorey, 1997; Siegel, Raveis, & Gorey,
    1998
Schrimshaw & Siegel, 2002; Siegel & Schrimshaw, 2000

Identical Reports

Walker, 1996, 1998

Positive Prenatal Diagnosis Studies

Published Reports

Alteneder, R. R., Kenner, C., Greene, D., & Pohorecki, S. (1998). The lived expe-
    rience of women who undergo prenatal diagnostic testing due to elevated
    maternal serum alpha-fetoprotein screening. MCN: *American Journal of
    Maternal-Child Nursing, 23,* 180–186.
Bryar, S. H. (1997). One day you're pregnant and one day you're not: Pregnancy
    interruption for fetal anomalies. JOGNN: *Journal of Obstetric, Gynecologic,
    & Neonatal Nursing, 26,* 559–566.
Furlong, R. M., & Black, R. B. (1984). Pregnancy termination for genetic indica-
    tions: The impact on families. *Social Work in Health Care, 10,* 17–34.

Helm, D. T., Miranda, S., & Chedd, N. A. (1998). Prenatal diagnosis of Down Syndrome: Mothers' reflections on supports needed from diagnosis to birth. *Mental Retardation, 36,* 55–61.

Kolker, A., & Burke, B. M. (1993). Grieving the wanted child: Ramifications of abortion after prenatal diagnosis of abnormality. *Health Care for Women International, 14,* 513–526.

Matthews, A. L. (1990). Known fetal malformations during pregnancy: A human experience of loss. *Birth Defects: Original Article Series, 26,* 168–175.

Rapp, R. (1988). The power of "positive" diagnosis: Medical and maternal discourses on amniocentesis. In K. L. Michaelson (Ed.), *Childbirth in America: Anthropological perspectives* (pp. 103–116). South Hadley, MA: Bergin & Garvey.

Rapp, R. (2000). *Testing women, testing the fetus: The social impact of amniocentesis in America.* New York: Routledge.

Redlinger-Grosse, K., Bernhardt, B. A., Berg, K., Muenke, M., & Biesecker, B. B. (2002). The decision to continue: The experiences and needs of parents who receive a prenatal diagnosis of holoprosencephaly. *American Journal of Medical Genetics, 112,* 369–378.

Rillstone, P., & Hutchinson, S. A. (2001). Managing the reemergence of anguish: Pregnancy after a loss due to anomalies. *JOGNN: Journal of Obstetric, Gynecologic, & Neonatal Nursing, 30,* 291–298.

Rothman, B. K. (1986). *The tentative pregnancy: Prenatal diagnosis and the future of motherhood.* New York: Viking.

Sandelowski, M., & Jones, L. C. (1996a). Couples' evaluations of foreknowledge of fetal impairment. *Clinical Nursing Research, 5,* 81–96.

Sandelowski, M., & Jones, L. C. (1996b). "Healing fictions": Stories of choosing in the aftermath of the detection of fetal anomalies. *Social Science & Medicine, 42,* 353–361.

Unpublished Reports

Menary, J. E. (1987). *The amniocentesis-abortion experience: A study of psychological effects and healing process.* Unpublished doctoral dissertation, Harvard University, Cambridge, MA.

Oustifine, J. M. (1990). *Abortion after amniocentesis: Women's lived experiences.* Unpublished Master's thesis, MGH Institute of Health Professions, Boston, MA.

Rillstone, P. (1999). *Prenatal diagnosis of fetal abnormalities: Managing catastrophic psychic pain in a subsequent pregnancy.* Unpublished doctoral dissertation, University of Florida, Gainesville.

Vantine, H. S. (2000). *Terminating a wanted pregnancy after the discovery of possible fetal abnormalities: An existential phenomenological study of making and living with the decision.* Unpublished doctoral dissertation, Duquesne University, Pittsburgh, PA.

POSITIVE PRENATAL DIAGNOSIS REPORTS
WITH IDENTICAL OR SHARED SAMPLES

Identical Samples

Rillstone 1999; Rillstone & Hutchinson, 2001
Sandelowski & Jones, 1996a, b

Shared Samples

Rapp, 1988, 2000

Index